Community-Based Research on LGBT Aging

The study of LGBT aging is in its infancy. In the absence of federal data on this often hidden population, community groups and organizations from across the country have taken it upon themselves to understand and assess the needs of this first cohort to reach later life in a time of LGBT public consciousness.

Eight papers are included in this compilation: three from the east coast (Boston, New York, and Washington, DC), four from the Midwest (Chicago, Bowling Green and surrounding areas, St. Louis, and the twin cities of Minneapolis/St. Paul), and one from the west coast (Palm Springs area). Together, these reports provide a community-based and regionally nuanced image of the strengths of, and the challenges faced by, older LGBT persons—local snapshots that together form a partial tapestry of LGBT aging in the U.S. They also serve as a source of lessons learned in the field—efforts that may be seen to parallel those undertaken by LGBT communities, then forming, during the 1980s and 1990s to address the growing health crisis of HIV/AIDS, a time when formal responses were slow and treatments still being developed. As such, the voice of the communities represented herein—the voices of these older adults—is clear, strong and apparent.

This book was originally published as a special issue of the *Journal of Homosexuality*.

Brian de Vries is professor of Gerontology at San Francisco State University, California, USA. He has authored or co-authored over 90 articles or chapters on issues including LGBT aging; he has edited or co-edited 4 books. He is a fellow of the Gerontological Society of America and former co-Chair of the LGBT Aging Issues Network of the American Society on Aging.

Catherine F. Croghan is a geriatric community health consultant and public health nurse. She frequently publishes and speaks on topics related to elder health and safety and has served on the American Society of Aging's LGBT Aging Issues Network Leadership Council and the National LGBT Aging Resource Centre's Advisory Council. Catherine co-founded Training to Serve, a Minnesota-based non-profit organisation that trains service providers to help them build skills for working with LGBT older adults.

Community-Based Research on LGBT Aging

Edited by
Brian de Vries and Catherine Croghan

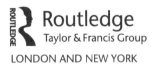
LONDON AND NEW YORK

First published 2015
by Routledge
2 Park Square, Milton Park, Abingdon, Oxfordshire OX14 4RN

and by Routledge
711 Third Avenue, New York, NY 10017, USA

First issued in paperback 2017

Routledge is an imprint of the Taylor & Francis Group, an informa business

© 2015 Taylor & Francis

British Library Cataloguing in Publication Data
A catalogue record for this book is available from the British Library

ISBN 13: 978-1-138-05801-9 (pbk)

ISBN 13: 978-1-138-85683-7 (hbk)

Typeset in ITC Garamond
by RefineCatch Limited, Bungay, Suffolk

Publisher's Note
The publisher accepts responsibility for any inconsistencies that may have arisen during the conversion of this book from journal articles to book chapters, namely the possible inclusion of journal terminology.

Disclaimer
Every effort has been made to contact copyright holders for their permission to reprint material in this book. The publishers would be grateful to hear from any copyright holder who is not here acknowledged and will undertake to rectify any errors or omissions in future editions of this book.

Contents

Part III: Interventions/Applications

Citation Information

The chapters in this book were originally published in the *Journal of Homosexuality*, volume 61, issue 1 (March 2014). When citing this material, please use the original page numbering for each article, as follows:

Chapter 1: Introduction
LGBT Aging: The Contributions of Community-Based Research
Brian de Vries and Catherine F. Croghan
Journal of Homosexuality, volume 61, issue 1 (March 2014) pp. 1–20

Chapter 2
Social Care Networks and Older LGBT Adults: Challenges for the Future
Mark Brennan-Ing, Liz Seidel, Britta Larson, and Stephen E. Karpiak
Journal of Homosexuality, volume 61, issue 1 (March 2014) pp. 21–52

Chapter 3
Investigating the Needs and Concerns of Lesbian, Gay, Bisexual, and Transgender Older Adults: The Use of Qualitative and Quantitative Methodology
Nancy A. Orel
Journal of Homosexuality, volume 61, issue 1 (March 2014) pp. 53–78

Chapter 4
Friends, Family, and Caregiving Among Midlife and Older Lesbian, Gay, Bisexual, and Transgender Adults
Catherine F. Croghan, Rajean P. Moone, and Andrea M. Olson
Journal of Homosexuality, volume 61, issue 1 (March 2014) pp. 79–102

Chapter 5
The Greater St. Louis LGBT Health and Human Services Needs Assessment: An Examination of the Silent and Baby Boom Generations
Meghan Jenkins Morales, M. Denise King, Hattie Hiler, Martin S. Coopwood, and Sherrill Wayland
Journal of Homosexuality, volume 61, issue 1 (March 2014) pp. 103–128

Chapter 6

Aging Out in the Desert: Disclosure, Acceptance, and Service Use Among Midlife and Older Lesbians and Gay Men
Aaron T. Gardner, Brian de Vries, and Danyte S. Mockus
Journal of Homosexuality, volume 61, issue 1 (March 2014) pp. 129–144

Chapter 7

Aging Out: A Qualitative Exploration of Ageism and Heterosexism Among Aging African American Lesbians and Gay Men
Imani Woody
Journal of Homosexuality, volume 61, issue 1 (March 2014) pp. 145–165

Chapter 8

Service Utilization Among Older Adults With HIV: The Joint Association of Sexual Identity and Gender
Mark Brennan-Ing, Liz Seidel, Andrew S. London, Sean Cahill, and Stephen E. Karpiak
Journal of Homosexuality, volume 61, issue 1 (March 2014) pp. 166–196

Chapter 9

Do LGBT Aging Trainings Effectuate Positive Change in Mainstream Elder Service Providers?
Kristen E. Porter and Lisa Krinsky
Journal of Homosexuality, volume 61, issue 1 (March 2014) pp. 197–216

Please direct any queries you may have about the citations to clsuk.permissions@cengage.com

Notes on Contributors

Mark Brennan-Ing is Director for Research and Evaluation at the AIDS Community Research Initiative of America, ACRIA Centre on HIV & aging, New York City, New York, USA. He also currently serves as an Adjunct Professor at the New York University College of Nursing.

Sean Cahill is Director of Health Policy Research at the Fenway Institute, Boston, Massachusetts, USA, where he focuses on LGBT health and HIV policy. Since 2010 he has served as an Adjunct Assistant Professor of Public Administration at the Robert Wagner School of Public Service, New York University, USA.

Martin S. Coopwood is Facilities Surveyor at the Missouri Department of Health and Senior Services, St. Louis, Missouri, USA.

Catherine F. Croghan is based at Croghan Consulting, Roseville, Minnesota, USA.

Brian de Vries is Professor in the Gerontology program at San Francisco State University, San Francisco, California, USA.

Aaron T. Gardner is a Research Specialist for the Department of Public Health, Riverside County, California, USA.

Hattie Hiler is based at Sage Metro St. Louis, St. Louis, Missouri, USA.

Stephen E. Karpiak is Senior Director for Research & Evaluation at the AIDS Community Research Initiative of America, ACRIA Centre on HIV & aging, New York City, New York, USA.

M. Denise King is Assistant Professor in the Department of Social Work, Lindenwood University, St. Charles, Missouri, USA.

Lisa Krinsky is Director of the LGBT Aging Project at the Fenway Institute, Boston, Massachusetts, USA.

Britta Larson is Senior Services Director at Center on Halsted, Chicago, Illinois, USA.

Andrew S. London is Chair of the Department of Sociology and Senior Research Associate at the Centre for Policy Research at Syracuse University, New York, USA.

Danyte S. Mockus is an Epidemiologist for the Department of Public Health, Riverside County, California, USA.

Rajean P. Moone is Executive Director of Training to Service, St. Paul, Minnesota, USA.

Meghan Jenkins Morales is the Manager of Benefits, Information and Education at AgeOptions, Oak Park, Illinois, USA.

Andrea M. Olson is Associate Professor of Psychology at St. Catherine University, St. Paul, Minnesota, USA.

Nancy A. Orel is Professor in the Gerontology programme at Bowling Green State University, Bowling Green, Ohio, USA.

Kristen E. Porter is based in the Department of Gerontology at the University of Massachusetts, Boston, Massachusetts, USA.

Liz Seidel is Manager for Research and Evaluation at the AIDS Community Research Initiative of America, ACRIA Centre on HIV & aging, New York City, New York, USA.

Sherrill Wayland is Executive Director at Sage Metro St. Louis, St. Louis, Missouri, USA.

Imani Woody is President and CEO of Mary's House for Older Adults, Inc., Washington, DC, USA.

INTRODUCTION

LGBT Aging: The Contributions of Community-Based Research

BRIAN de VRIES, PhD

Gerontology Program, San Francisco State University, San Francisco, California, USA

CATHERINE F. CROGHAN, MS, MPH, RN

Croghan Consulting, Roseville, Minnesota, USA

Lesbian, gay, bisexual, and transgender (LGBT) aging, as a field of research and as a focus of public interest, has witnessed dramatic growth in the past few years. As de Vries and Herdt (2011) have noted, it was only a few decades ago that the terms *aging* and *LGBT* were thought to be, at best, incongruous and, at worst, incompatible. In the intervening years, and most recently in the past decade, LGBT aging has been highlighted in numerous publications and books, addressed within the Institute of Medicine (IOM; 2011) report on LGBT health, been the focus of recent efforts within the Department of Health and Human Services and the National Institutes of Health, and benefitted from the impressive expansion of SAGE (Services and Advocacy for GLBT Elders) through a network of affiliates around the United States, as well as numerous community-based service organizations. Much has been learned through and based on these many efforts—even as many questions remain unexplored, and many issues remained unaddressed.

In the absence of any federal data specifically addressing sexual orientation and gender identity, the research that exists is largely based on smaller availability samples (with some impressive exceptions) with studies often conducted (and often funded) by community organizations. These actions may be seen to parallel those undertaken by LGBT communities, then forming, during the 1980s and 1990s to address the growing health crisis of HIV/AIDS. In these dark years, thousands of lives were lost to this disease at first not yet named and later strongly associated with gay men.

At a time when governments shamefully turned their backs on those in the most dire health circumstances, a community responded; lesbians and bisexual women, gay and bisexual men, and transgender women and men came together as rarely before and rose to the challenge of care when many others retreated. They formed networks of care and created services, and in the process solidified a community and developed a political presence. Extensions of those earlier efforts are those now being directed toward issues related to LGBT older adults and are the basis of this special issue.

Contemporary community groups, in the absence of federal data and broader network attention, appreciation, and comprehension, have taken it upon themselves to understand and assess the needs of this first cohort to reach later life in a time of LGBT public consciousness. Older LGBT persons have few models to direct their actions and offer support; older LGBT adults have witnessed the loss of many of their colleagues and friends with whom they expected to grow old—their systems of support often identified "chosen families." Services provided for older adults often fail to recognize the unique circumstances of LGBT aging. Many community groups have not failed to recognize this need and many of their efforts are reported herein.

This special issue of the *Journal of Homosexuality* is focused on LGBT aging and informed by some of the many community-based needs assessments and studies conducted throughout the United States. The publication of these efforts is intended to provide a community-based image of older LGBT persons—local snapshots that together form a partial quilt or tapestry of LGBT aging in the United States. Often, the intention of the groups conducting these studies was not to publish the results, but purely to understand a need to which they could respond. As such, effort has been expended to render these reports in the language of empirical social science. But, the voice of the community—the voices of these older adults—remains clear, strong, and apparent.

This article serves to introduce these reports and set the stage for this special issue. In the text that follows, a brief introduction to each of the articles is offered. This is followed by a review of some of their findings, placed in the context of the existing literature on LGBT. The findings in these community-based reports reinforce some of those from the burgeoning literature and also provide a new and deeper context for their interpretation, and addressing both what communities want to know and often what the existing literature has not yet addressed. More important, in their aggregate, these articles and these findings further highlight the diversity within the LGBT communities and help deepen our understanding, setting the stage for more complex and complete examinations of this population and better-tailored programming; they provide a more nuanced understanding of the lives and circumstances of LGBT aging.

Similarly, just as much may be learned from the results of these studies, so, too, is there much to learn from the conduct of this research. These community groups have often stretched themselves in unfamiliar ways to make sure this research has taken place; there are lessons to be told about how research in the LGBT community is most appropriately and productively done. There are lessons to be told about the role of research in community-based activities and programming, also reviewed here. This issue stands as evidence of a field unfolding, of communities caring and responding, and of varying paths to and experiences of later life—the understanding of which benefits all.

COMMUNITY-BASED NEEDS ASSESSMENTS

This special issue of the *Journal of Homosexuality* presents a series of articles that have their base in community-based assessments of the needs, concerns, and issues of LGBT aging and older persons. Eight empirical articles comprise this special issue that offer quantitative and qualitative work, in communities larger and smaller, from Massachusetts to the California desert. Together, the experiences of over 2,800 LGBT persons are represented in some form.

Three articles help to frame the issues, and offer fresh perspectives on the same. Mark Brennan-Ing, Liz Seidel, Britta Larson, and Stephen E. Karpiak (2014/this issue) present the findings from an in-depth assessment of the social needs of 210 LGBT older adults in Chicago, through the Center on Halstead, finding high levels of need, particularly in the area of socialization, with networks of support that are disproportionately friend-based—that is, persons of comparable age and need. Nancy A. Orel (2014/this issue) presents findings from three studies, some preliminary, some qualitative ($N = 75$ over 2 studies) and some quantitative ($N = 1,150$), exploring the needs of LGBT elders with samples from northern Ohio and southeastern Michigan; highlighting a multi-method approach to studying these complex issues, she also introduces a particular focus on gay and lesbian grandparents, one of many understudied populations whose experiences are made more complex by generational views of homosexuality and the mediating role of the parents. Catherine F. Croghan, Rajean P. Moone, and Andrea M. Olson (2014/this issue) present the most recent of studies analyzing data from a large sample ($N = 495$) in the Twin Cities area of Minnesota; with a particular focus on caregiving, they find that LGBT older adults are less likely to have traditional sources of caregiver support and are more likely to be serving as a caregiver and caring for someone to whom they were not legally related, with all the uncertainty that entails.

Four articles build on this foundation and highlight the diversity within LGBT populations and settings. Meghan Jenkins Morales, M. Denise King, Hattie Hiler, Martin S. Coopwood, and Sherrill Wayland (2014/this issue) examine the generational-specific and shared needs of 151 LGBT older persons in the St. Louis area of Missouri. Aaron T. Gardner, Brian de Vries, and Danyte S. Mockus (2014/this issue), examine the roles of gender and age in levels of disclosure, social service use, and acceptance among LGBT persons in the second half of life and beyond. This study of 502 lesbians and gay men, primarily from the California desert city of Palm Springs, reveals that older lesbians fear being open about their sexual orientation more so than do men and, concomitantly, believe acceptance in their chosen communities and recognition within the organizations that provide services to older adults is important. Imani Woody (2014/this issue) addresses the needs of an older sample of 15 African American gay men and lesbians in the Washington, DC area, highlighting the sometimes overlapping, sometimes competing effects of racial and sexual orientation stigma on the experiences of aging. Mark Brennan-Ing, Liz Seidel, Andrew S. London, Sean Cahill, and Stephen E. Karpiak (2014/this issue) present an analysis of the service use of 180 older persons with HIV accessing services from the Gay Men's Health Crisis in New York City; they report a strong form of accelerated aging, in a context of weak social support, with few differences between gay, lesbian, bisexual and heterosexual older adults—HIV serves to render aging experiences comparable and hastened.

A final article, by Kristen E. Porter and Lisa Krinsky (2014/this issue), explores the efficacy of trainings provided by the Boston LGBT Aging Project to 76 mainstream social service providers about LGBT aging, revealing a variety of erroneous assumptions with some implicit negative attitudes on the part of service providers; their study shows how an educational intervention can generate change in both.

In the following section, some of the central findings of these reports are summarized and placed in the context of existing research on LGBT aging. In so doing, the impressive contributions offered by these articles are highlighted along with a snapshot of what has been previously reported in the field. Several themes organize this burgeoning literature; these include a focus on the demographics of the population (e.g., socioeconomic status, relationship status, disclosure and identity), social support (including a focus on friendship and families of choice as well the offering and receipt of care), health and wellbeing (including both physical and psychological health), and the pervasive role of stigma (as reflected earlier). These themes structure the following review.

LGBT AGING RESEARCH: A REVIEW AND SUMMARY

Demographics

Estimating the numbers of LGBT persons is a difficult task (for reasons of stigma, variability in definitions and terms, and malleability over time and circumstance, among other reasons) with varying political, empirical, and social consequences. For those over the age of 65, this could represent four or more million people, but without solid, federal data, these will remain estimates at best (Movement Advancement Project, 2010). The addition of the baby boomer cohort may easily double these numbers.

One source of variability in the accounting of this population derives from the terms used in self-description. For example, Adelman, Gurevitch, de Vries, and Blando (2006) found, with a sample of just over 1,300 LGBT people ranging in ages from 18 to 92, that, although most women who have sex with women (WSW) identify as "lesbian," older (i.e., ages 65 and older) women are much more likely (by a factor of almost 10) to identify as "gay" than are younger women. Examining men from the same study, the differences are more modest, yet still evocative. Men who have sex with men (MSM) ages 65 and older are much more likely to identify as "homosexual" (about $1\frac{1}{2}$ times more likely) and less likely to identify as "gay" (about one-third less likely) than men in other age groups (something also noted by Rawls, 2004). Although not significant in these analyses, younger men also were more likely to identify as "queer" than were men in the middle and later years. This signals an interesting discrepancy in self-reference by age group and perhaps poses one of the well-known hurdles that exist in the promotion of intergenerational LGBT ties.

Woody's contribution to this special issue adds important further dimensionality to this subject; in her qualitative research with lesbians and gay men of color, she finds a marked distaste for terms like gay and lesbian, among the range of terms often used. Respondents in her sample describe a preference for more relational terms (e.g., "same-gender loving"), which she reports may be cohort-based or influenced by culture and race.

Related to the terms used is the extent to which an individual is "out" or guarded about her or his identity. In a national sample of LGBT boomers (i.e., those ages 45–64), significant differences were noted on this dimension (MetLife, 2010). Guardedness (i.e., being less "out") decreased with the intimacy of the relationship; that is, LGBT persons were more guarded with neighbors than they were with other family and than they were with siblings. Most prominent in these data, however, was the extent to which transgender and especially bisexual women and men were guarded than were gay men and lesbians, across settings. This guardedness extends to health care settings as well, an important issue is securing sensitive and personal health care. Even among their closest friends, over 30% of bisexual boomers but did not identify as such. The costs and consequences of such guardedness are an important area to pursue.

The level of "outness" was considered by several of the studies in this journal issue; Orel included a modified scale of measuring openness and outness—a measure more complex than most and notes association between disclosure and service use; Jenkins Morales et al. reported significant age and cohort differences in outness, with those among the young-old more likely to report being "out" than those among the older-old, something also implicit in the findings of Gardner et al. and replicating previous research. Gender differences emerged in the Gardner et al. article, however, not typically reported in previous research, with women expressing greater concern about being accepted as a member of a sexual or gender minority in their chosen community and, in comparable fashion, more likely to feel comfortable using services that identified as LGBT in some form. These authors suggest the role of the gendered context and distribution as one potential interpretation of this evocative finding.

There remains a persistent myth of the relative affluence of an LGBT population notwithstanding a fairly substantial body of data noting that LGBT persons, and perhaps especially older adults, have somewhat lower incomes than comparably aged heterosexual persons (Badgett, 2002). This has been reported in both local and national studies. Interestingly, LGBT adults tend to be more highly educated, however (also supported by a wide array of both national and local studies), and several of the contributions to this special issue echo these results: Brennan-Ing, Seidel, Larson, and Karpiak; Croghan et al.; Jenkins Morales et al.; and Woody. Together, these findings provide an unexpected point of contrast to the frequently noted association between income and education; this relationship appears to be dramatically weakened in the LGBT populations studied.

Perhaps one of the most consistent findings across studies, both national studies where they exist and more often local research, is that LGBT older adults are much more likely than are heterosexual and non-transgender adults to be single (not partnered) and without children (e.g., IOM, 2011). In San Francisco Bay Area data (Adelman et al., 2006), for example, almost 75% of gay men aged 65 and older and about one-half of lesbians of comparable ages identified themselves as single; interestingly, although not surprisingly, about the same percentages reported that they did not have any children. In a national study of over 1,200 LGBT boomers (MetLife, 2010), with a comparison sample of comparable size from the general population, it was found that LGBT persons were more than $1\frac{1}{2}$ times more likely to be single than the predominantly heterosexual population. About 12% of gay male boomers were single, never in a relationship—a percentage that is at least 4 times higher than heterosexual men, as well as women both lesbian and heterosexual. At the same time, recent data reveal that older gay men are 3 times more likely to live alone than are heterosexual older men and are one-half as likely to live with a partner; the differences between lesbians and heterosexual women is more modest (Wallace, Cochran, Durazo, & Ford, 2011).

Research reported in this compilation similarly find that older gay men are significantly less likely to be partnered in some form (Brennan-Ing, Seidel, Larson, & Karpiak, 2014/this issue; Croghan et al., 2014/this issue; and Jenkins Morales et al., 2014/this issue), more likely to be single (Brennan-Ing,

Seidel, Larson, & Karpiak, 2014/this issue; Croghan et al., 2014/this issue), and are more likely to live alone (Brennan-Ing, Seidel, Larson, & Karpiak, 2014/this issue; Croghan et al., 2014/this issue). In their study on older persons with HIV, Brennan-Ing, Seidel, London, et al. (2014/this issue) found that almost three-fourths of their sample of primarily men lived alone. Croghan et al. also note that gay men are less likely to have children (than most other sexual orientation groups). Given the well substantiated principle of substitution noted in the Gerontology field (Cantor & Mayer, 1978; wherein elders are seen to first turn to their spouse, then adult children, and then other family for care when needs arise), this finding particularly places LGBT older adults (and perhaps gay men in particular) at increased risk of having unmet medical and social needs. Interestingly, Croghan et al. also note that bisexual men and women and transgender women were significantly *more* likely to have children than were other sexual orientation and gender identity groups. These same researchers report that transgender women were also most likely to live with a partner. These findings add further dimensionality to the research and understanding of age-based relational ties and sexual orientation and gender identity; these findings merit further investigation and consideration.

Social Support

In the absence of conventional family support systems, upon which policy is often predicated, LGBT persons have come to place a high value on their friendships (e.g., de Vries & Megathlin, 2009), what some authors have called "families of choice," or "logical kin" as a contrast to "biological kin" (to quote Armistead Maupin, 2007). In several large studies, it has been found that LGBT older adults identify a greater number of friends than do comparably aged heterosexual persons (e.g., MetLife, 2010). In the MetLife study of LGBT baby-boomers, almost two-thirds of respondents said that they had a "family of choice"; a high proportion of LGBT boomers also said that they would turn to these friends for a wide variety of needs (e.g., support or encouragement, errands, and emergency), as well as offer friends such care—proportions that were much higher than those of the general population (MetLife, 2010).

Particularly following the onset of HIV/AIDS and the initial federal and often state non-response to the crisis, LGBT people sought and found each other, creating services to meet the special needs and, in the process, creating a sense of community (albeit broad and somewhat diffuse), as noted earlier. Such relations, however, fall outside of typical policy and program parameters with a focus on family ties and obligations for care provision: Friends are not expected to be, and often not respected as, caregivers (Barker, 2002). Moreover, friends (mostly of comparable age) may not be able or available to provide the care that is needed by an LGBT elder. This precarious social support has been frequently noted in both the descriptive and empirical research literatures; this precariousness has particular dramatic implications when one considers the increasing need for support that may accompany age.

Further depth to the understanding of this area is provided by several of the articles in this journal issue. Croghan et al., for example, found about two-thirds of their sample of LGBT persons over the age of 48 reported that they had "enough close friends"; bisexual women reporting significantly higher percentages. These friends are the likely constituents of "chosen families" and almost three-fourths of Croghan et al.'s sample identified a family of choice; interestingly, bisexual men differed from the other groups, with about one-half saying they had a family of choice. Brennan-Ing, Seidel, Larson, and Karpiak reported that their social networks (the association of these networks to chosen families remains to be more fully explored) comprised about 10 people, at least 4 of whom were friends. Women identified larger networks than did men, perhaps attributable to their inclusion of children and other family members. Still, as reported by Jenkins Morales et al., the majority of older LGBT respondents felt that they at least sometimes lacked companionship; these authors also reported that loneliness was negatively related to identity disclosure and positively related to perceived barriers to health care. Woody notes the important (and understudied) role of race; African American older gay men and lesbians discussed a pervasive sense of alienation—from the African American community, from their religion, and even within the LGBT community. These findings suggest many profitable and meaningful avenues for future research (with policy implications) on the impact of race, gender, and sexual orientation on social support.

In terms of caregiving, Croghan et al. (2014/this issue) note that the majority of their respondents report that they have someone to look after them if they were to become ill, although the person most identified was the partner (and previously mentioned research suggests that large numbers of LGBT persons are without partners—especially men). Friends were mentioned second in frequency for both anticipated caregiver and likely care-recipient. Encouragingly, within this context, Brennan-Ing, Seidel, Larson, and Karpiak (2014/this issue) find that help from friends was not significantly different from help from family. They further appropriately distinguish between positive and negative support (given that not all support attempts are necessarily helpful) and find a higher proportion of negative support from family than from friends. Clearly, this is an area prime for further investigation, given the demographic characteristics of this population and the findings in this area, nuanced by the reports of this special issue.

Health and Wellbeing

Later life may bring with it some particular physical and mental health issues for an LGBT aging population—in addition to all that accompanies later life more generally. In general, and based on research with national samples with comparison samples from the general population, LGBT persons are more likely to report that their general health is poor (Massachusetts Department of Public Health, 2009). The poorer health is associated with higher rates of some cancers (anal cancers for gay men and higher rates of exposure to human papillomavirus: Chin-Hong et al., 2004; reproductive cancers for lesbians: Valanis et al., 2000) and of disabilities (47%, with rates for women higher than rates for men; Fredriksen-Goldsen et al., 2011). Asthma and Diabetes are also seen more frequently among LGBT persons than among the general population (Adelman et al., 2006); there are also higher rates of HIV/AIDS (Fredriksen-Goldsen et al., 2011).

The articles by Brennan-Ing, Seidel, Larson, and Karpiak and Brennan-Ing, Seidel, London, et al. included in this special issue speak directly to these health conditions and implications, echoing some of the findings and adding specificity, particularly in the context of HIV/AIDS. In the Brennan-Ing, Seidel, London, et al. examination of the service use of midlife and older persons with HIV, they find considerable consistency in the nature of needs, and of experiences, across sexual orientation and gender, although older gay men were somewhat more likely to have a diagnosis of AIDS than were men and women in other sexual orientation groups. Overall, the experience of aging with HIV/AIDS is associated with higher rates of age-associated illnesses, often decades prior to when they might be expected. Older persons with HIV/AIDS also live with an average of 3.4 additional health conditions, further challenging their quality of life and experience of aging. A surprisingly comparable number of chronic health conditions (i.e., 3) was also noted in the Chicago study of social care among LGBT older persons in general by Brennan-Ing, Seidel, Larson, and Karpiak. About 30% of the respondents in this study also reported that they were disabled. The role of HIV was also noted in this study: About one-fourth of the friends identified by older LGBT persons, with higher proportions among gay men, were HIV-positive—returning to the precariousness of these networks amidst an elevated need for care.

Compounding these high rates of disabilities and some diseases, LGBT older adults are less likely to have health insurance and more likely to delay seeking health care (and related services, including screenings and prescriptions)—and, although studies are few and rare, these findings appear to be particularly true for transgender older adults (Movement Advancement Project, 2010). It is worth noting that the contributions by Jenkins Morales et al. (2014/this issue) and Brennan-Ing, Seidel, Larson, and Karpiak (2014/this issue) point to high levels of midlife and older LGBT persons with health insurance, although the fact that many are eligible for, and recipients of, Medicare certainly plays a role in this. Seven percent of the sample described by Brennan-Ing, Seidel, Larson, and Karpiak in Chicago received health care from Veterans' Affairs; 13% had served in the military.

These proportions suggest an avenue of research, LGBT (aging) and the military, that is just opening.

LGBT adults have been noted to have higher rates of smoking (especially lesbians; Gruskin, Greenwood, Matevia, Pollack, & Bye, 2007; Tang et al., 2004); there are also reports of more problem drinking (somewhat more commonly noted among older lesbians than gay men; Grossman, D'Augelli, & O'Connell, 2001; Valanis et al., 2000). Dramatically, LGBT older adults have high rates of exposure to violence and victimization over course of lives (higher for men than for women and even higher for transgender persons; D'Augelli & Grossman, 2001; Fredriksen-Goldsen et al., 2011). These may be both exacerbating circumstances of some of the previously mentioned diseases and related to poorer health screening and other public health interventions.

The article by Jenkins Morales et al. (2014/this issue) specifically address experiences of violence, victimization, and abuse with dramatic frequency and variations attributable to age, gender, and gender identity. For example, almost two-thirds (61.6%) of the older adults in this study report having experienced some form of homophobic violence or victimization over the lifetimes; almost 58% have experienced verbal harassment, with rates higher for men than for women and with younger older adults reporting higher rates of harassment than those older.

Related to the violence and victimization just noted, LGBT persons are also at risk of greater psychological and emotional distress—that is, LGBT older adults report depression at higher rates (more than $2\frac{1}{2}$ times higher than the general population for gay men and more than $1\frac{1}{2}$ times higher for lesbians; Mills et al., 2004). Along comparable lines, high rates of suicidal thoughts and behaviors have also been noted, almost 3 times higher for gay and bisexual men and almost 2 times higher for lesbian and bisexual women (data inclusive of, but not restricted to, older adults; Balsam, Rothblum, & Beauchaine, 2005).

Support for and depth to these findings is again introduced by the work reported herein. Brennan-Ing, Seidel, Larson, and Karpiak (2014/this issue) similarly found that gay men report depression at higher rates than other groups. Depression rates were substantial and comparable (around 16%) in the sample described by Jenkins Morales et al. (2014/this issue), who also noted that those older adults with probable depression were also more likely to have experienced homophobic violence and victimization and were more likely to perceive barriers to health care. Among older persons with HIV/AIDS, at least moderate depression was reported by more than 50% of the sample, with 35% reporting a level of symptoms on the Center for Epidemiological Studies–Depression Scale indicative of severe depression (Radloff, 1977).

Clearly, there are physical and psychological conditions that distinguish LGBT aging; many of these circumstances that give rise to these physical conditions may be rooted in the experiences of stigma, sadly common in the lives of LGBT persons.

Stigma

LGBT persons, as is true of everyone, live lives shaped by history. The popularization of the term "cohort," as seen in references to "the greatest generation" and the "boomers," draws attention to these temporal and cultural influences on aging. But, today's older LGBT population matured and developed during times when their expressions of love were "diagnosed" as a psychiatric disorder (which was eliminated from the *Diagnostic and Statistical Manual of Mental Disorders* only in 1973 [American Psychiatric Association, 1973]) and whose committed relationships, even today, are the subject of intense debate with ongoing experiences and threats of constitutional exclusion in the United States. These are individuals who, through the course of their lives, have been labeled as sick, immoral, illegal, and unnatural (e.g., Kochman, 1997); these are women and men who endured and have seen AIDS decimate their social networks and destroy their communities. These historical markers certainly have left an imprint.

These experiences of stigma are not just historical, however. A recent report notes that even today almost 80% of older LGBT persons feel that they cannot be "out" in long-term care settings; over 80% of their caregivers and other service providers feel the same (National Senior Citizens Law Center, 2011). Almost the same percentage fear discrimination by staff and other residents in long-term care settings, and almost one-half fear abuse or neglect.

Stigma in many ways serves as an organizing construct unifying the findings and experiences reviewed earlier—that is, stigma may well underlie the mental, and even physical and demographic effects noted earlier—part of a generalized stress with which LGBT persons live and age (Meyer, 2003), which, like a weight, LGBT people carry with them over the course of their daily lives—with costs and consequences. Psychological distress may be seen as a natural consequence of stigma; the broader lack of recognition of same-sex relationships may be said to have led to the development of non-traditional relationships and a prominent focus on non-kin ties (even as these friends and other non-relatives are often failed to be recognized by social and health institutions caring for an LGBT person). This lack of recognition has a pronounced effect on income and access to resources in later life (Herdt & Kertzner, 2006). Recent research has found that when relationships are not recognized, LGBT boomers (of all relationship statuses) are more likely to fear discrimination and treatment in later life (de Vries, Mason, Quam, & Acquaviva, 2009). Similarly, a study published in 2012 found that legal marriage is associated with health benefits for same-sex couples above and beyond even domestic partnerships (Wight, LeBlanc, de Vries, & Detels, 2012). Studies have shown that safety net programs and laws intended to support and protect older Americans fail to provide equal protections for LGBT elders. For example, limitations on the opportunities for same-sex couples to marry have an impact on their eligibility to receive the benefits of Social Security and Medicare, among others similar inequalities may be noted among retirement plans, health insurance benefits, and a wide array of taxes (Herek, 2006).

The studies included in this special issue similarly speak to the ongoing fears and stress that accompany the aging of LGBT populations in a heteronormative and frequently unaccepting environment. The dramatic reports of abuse, violence, and victimization certainly attest to this. Moreover, all of the studies, in some form, identify socialization needs of older LGBT people—a desire to be among "one's own people" with concomitant reduced anxieties and shared perspectives and reduced need to conceal integral parts of a person's identity, as Woody particularly and poignantly noted. Most of the studies point to the need for LGBT affirmative social and health services to afford respectful and sensitive care and treatment. Orel reported that 53% of her large Midwest sample felt that existing services did not meet the unique needs of LGB older adults; 42% reported negative experiences with health care attributable to sexual orientation and gender identity. The evaluation research study of Porter and Krinsky addresses this issue specifically. They find that even in an urban center, even within organizations that have the awareness of LGBT aging issues to seek training, and even with organizations that have LGBT employees, a brief educational intervention resulted in increased awareness of LGBT resources, the many policy disparities that affect LGBT elders, as well as factual knowledge about the lives of older LGBT persons and the discrimination they face.

These experiences of exclusion, separateness, and lack of recognition also may be seen, however, to be associated with a greater self-reliance as a way of "doing for oneself" when others have failed to do so. Several authors (e.g., Kimmel, 1978) have proposed that LGBT older adults have fashioned a sense of hardiness and competence out of a lifetime of surviving as a sexual or gender minority in a heterosexual environment—a strategy of engaging their environment that may bode well for success in the challenges of later life (de Vries, 2006). Almost three-fourths of the national sample of LGBT boomers reported that they thought being LGBT had helped prepare them for aging; interestingly, just over one-half also thought that being LGBT had made aging more difficult (MetLife, 2010). Perhaps being freed (or excluded) from the relative bounds of traditional gender role definitions have afforded LGBT persons the opportunity to engage in gender-incongruent behaviors throughout their lives that heterosexuals typically do not confront. Authors have come to frame such findings in the terms of "positive marginality" (Unger, 2000): the view that one's stigmatized characteristics may be a source of strength and that banding with those similarly stigmatized may provide a vehicle for social change.

Evidence of such adaptability and growth may similarly be seen in this special issue. Woody makes this point more directly; she reports that many of her respondents noted that the challenges they experienced based on racial or gender oppression made it easier to deal with oppression based on age. Many developed a sagacity through their experience of hostile environments over the course of their live. They commented that their "otherness" facilitated the opportunity to grow and nurture their networks of friends. Orel found similar results among a larger, diverse sample of LGBT older persons. Brennan-Ing, Seidel, Larson, and Karpiak also noted that many LGBT adults saw aging as a chance to grow, explore, and make the most of life. These experiences, and this range of experience in response to stigma, merits attention and offer an opportunity to observe and learn from the resilience of older LGBT people.

Diversity and LGBT Older Adults

The previous material presents a portrait of older LGBT persons in an increasingly varied context—from self-referent issues, to personal health and relationships, to social organizations and actions. Mounting research studies support the many challenges LGBT elders face and endure—and the strengths they bring to these encounters, for themselves and others. One observation about this burgeoning field is clear and probably without dissent: LGBT older adults are a diverse group of people.

As the IOM (2011) report noted, the acronym LGBT describes a broad coalition of groups comprising women and men (and those who shun either label), most homosexual, some bisexual, some heterosexual (about 25% of transgender boomers identify as straight; MetLife, 2010), and those who eschew any such label. Moreover, the groups under this umbrella term are further diverse with respect to race and ethnicity; socioeconomic status; geographic location; urban, rural, or in between; among myriad other characteristics. Age and cohort are certainly important such characteristics.

Age has often been described in the terms of a fan (where with increasing age comes increasing complexity and variability), so, too, may the description of LGBT aging be seen. The many sources of diversity inherent in the LGBT population in general are likely exacerbated among an older population of LGBT persons. Consider the samples described in the contributions of this special issue: In the aggregate, these LGBT older adults comprise women and men who are gay, bisexual, lesbian, or queer; Caucasian, African American, Latino, Asian or Pacific Islander, American Indian or Alaska Native, or multiracial/ethnic; in their middle and later years, from urban and rural settings, in "red" and "blue" states, who are single (through a variety of forces, including by choice, by circumstance, and through the death of loved ones) or partnered (in a variety of ways); live alone or with others in various settings; have varying educational backgrounds and varying levels of income (sufficiency); are parents and grandparents or neither; are "out" to varying degrees; are retired or employed full or part time; may or may not have served in the military; may or may not have a history of incarceration; are HIV-positive and HIV-negative; have varying degrees of health—mental and physical—disabilities and chronic conditions; and have varying degrees of religious investments. All of these conditions and circumstances are at least influenced by age and likely made more complex.

These factors, in combination, likely underscore several of the evocative findings of reported in the articles of this special issue that point to this diversity: the gender differences noted in Gardner et al. to which the authors draw our attention to the gendered and regional context within which studies take place; the racial context that Woody describes, serving to highlight settings that separate and settings that integrate; the role of health, particularly the role of HIV, as Brennan-Ing, Seidel, Larson, and Karpiak and Brennan-Ing, Seidel, London, et al. point out in their articles, with HIV implying important and potentially fragile network support (both needed and potentially available) and how HIV serves to diminish yet other differences (e.g., the comparability of other groups, both women and men, gay and straight); the particular contexts of transgender older adults, often overlooked in research (so much so that it has been referred to as "the silent 'T'"), wherein transgender women are more likely to be partnered also more likely to have children (at least more so than lesbians and gay men), as Croghan et al. point out; the particular experiences of grandparents, as Orel notes, as they navigate multiple roles and relationships outside of the scope of much prior research and theory; and the cohort differences among LGBT older adults that Jenkins Morales et al. address, something often overlooked in many fields. A comprehensive program to portray and understand LGBT elders necessarily includes many of these nuances; results of such programs lead to changes in attitudes, behaviors, and knowledge, as Porter and Krinsky point out.

A better understanding of the LGBT aging community, in all of its complexity and diversity, is not only the basis for effective and competent service provision to meet their needs, it mandates reflection on the assumptions underlying policies and services and provides an opportunity to reconsider how best to engage and work with an increasingly diverse older population (de Vries & Blando, 2004). Many of these issues have relevance to the lives of heterosexual older adults as well—that is, heterosexual couples may also enter old age without children, single, or in non-marital relationships; a close and family-like network of friends is not exclusive to LGBT persons; and independence is valued by most in the North American context. Policies and programs that address the effects of stigma include non-traditional family forms and honor diverse life trajectories have benefits for all. The research reported in this issue help point the way to the areas that merit further attention, the impact they may have, and how best to make use of these resources.

Several of these studies have been used in policy and program advances and these are reviewed later. Notwithstanding these many programmatic and empirical contributions, however, the studies included in this special issue are necessarily bracketed by samples and other limitations. It is important to both understand and underscore these potential limiting factors and these are also summarized later.

Limitations

Of the eight articles included in the special issue, six were conducted within a broader community setting, one surveyed clients in an AIDS service organization, and one surveyed staff at multiple service provider settings. All eight studies used convenience (availability) samples and noted difficulties in obtaining adequate gender identity, sexual orientation, or ethnic and racial diversity. The six broader-based community surveys recruited participants through LGBT community organizations; relied on "agents"—individuals with access to the LGBT community (with attendant strength and weaknesses)—to recruit participants; or used snowballing techniques, where individuals who completed the survey, then extended personal invitations to friends and acquaintances to do the same.

Of these methods, recruiting through community organizations was the most common approach. However, convenience or availability samples drawn in this manner are known to include individuals who are more "out" and socially connected—that is, these samples may have an overrepresentation of individuals who are comfortable enough with their sexual orientation or gender identities to be associated with an LGBT community organization.

None of the studies reported samples that drew large numbers of bisexual or transgender individuals. Most of the broader community survey samples had ethnic and racial profiles that did not match the general population or, if they did match, the numbers of non-White respondents were too low to allow analysis and further insight into the experiences of these populations. These sample problems suggest the need for research that targets the smaller populations within the LGBT community (e.g., bisexual men, Latina lesbians, and transgender men). Woody's article, "Aging Out," an exploration of African American gay men and lesbians in the Washington, DC area is an example of this approach. However, it too identifies the limitation of a small homogeneous sample that lacks geographic and socioeconomic diversity.

Other limitations spoke to the complexity of defining populations by sexual orientation or gender identity. Although terms such as lesbian, gay man, bisexual, and transgender might appear to define this population, many individuals identify outside these categories preferring queer or a variety of other identities—or eschewing any such label. Researchers working in the dynamic environment of sexual orientation and gender identity may find the evolution of definitions and identities make research design and analysis complex, as well as comparisons with past research more difficult (Quam & Croghan, 2008).

Not only are the identities within sexual orientation and gender identity dynamic, researchers also face a changing social environment where acceptance and legal protections may vary from state to state and month to month. Asking the relationship status of an individual and providing the options of spouse, partner, single or widow may sound straightforward, but the LGBT respondent who is legally married in one state and has moved to a state that does not recognize same-sex marriages, may not be sure how to answer this question. Is he a spouse? Similarly, the surviving partner of a long-term, but not legally recognized, relationship may not be certain if she is a widow.

Although all survey research calls for precision, the dynamic environment of LGBT culture and politics demands an added level of caution when constructing assessment tools and certainly suggests the need for a set of standard demographic measures that have been vetted for the very issues outlined here.

Contributors reported taking steps to use survey measures that would allow comparisons with prior LGBT research and the general population. The St. Louis study included in this special issue (Jenkins Morales et al., 2014/this issue) adapted a survey instrument used by Frazer (2009). The most recently completed survey (Croghan et al., 2014/this issue) included questions that allowed comparison with two recent national LGBT datasets (Fredriksen-Goldsen et al., 2011; MetLife, 2010), as well as regional data (Minnesota Board on Aging, 2005).

The IOM's (2011) compilation on LGBT health recommends the development and standardization of sexual orientation and gender identity measures. Adoption of standardized demographic questions, as well as a library of other content questions would allow clearer comparison of results from study to study and lead to a better understanding of the larger LGBT population.

Most of the initial LGBT community needs assessment were conducted with paper or hardcopy surveys, but more recent surveys are being made available either exclusively online or as a combination of online and paper surveys. Use of electronic survey tools greatly reduce the cost of conducting an assessment by eliminating the costs associated with printing, handling and mailing paper surveys, as well as subsequent data entry. However, they may well result in samples that over represent individuals with computer skills and greater Internet access perhaps also those with greater financial resources and education. However, because much of the community survey work is done by volunteers with little or no funding, or in service organizations with dwindling resources, it would appear methods will continue to shift toward less expensive online surveys.

APPLICATIONS OF COMMUNITY-BASED RESEARCH

Most surveys were conducted to develop local or regional information that would inform policy and assist program planners to better address the needs of a population that is not well understood. Jenkins Morales et al. (2014/this issue) describe this type of use in the St. Louis Area where results fostered a relationship with the local long-term care ombudsman program that in turn led to training of nursing home staff across the state on the needs of LGBT older adults. Results were also used to strengthen the recently formed SAGE Metro St. Louis affiliate and begin planning for the needs of LGBT baby boomers.

A few of the surveys included in this issue were conducted some time ago, such as the 2003 cultural competency training curriculum evaluation work reported by Porter and Krinsky, allowing for a discussion of how they have influenced a variety of outcomes in the ensuing years. The training evaluation they document led to adoption of the curriculum by the LGBT Aging Project's Open Door Task Force and the proliferation of service provider training within the region. Other surveys were completed more recently and have fewer outcomes to report. However, all make suggestions for how results might be used and outline future research questions that build on their findings. One of the more recent surveys, the LGBT Elders Needs Assessment Scale (Orel, 2014/this issue), is still open and preliminary analyses have already influenced further research. Initial data review suggested the development of a research project exploring the experiences of LGBT grandparents. That pilot study is currently underway.

Many communities have completed more than one survey. Croghan et al. (2014/this issue) build on earlier survey work (Croghan, Mertens, Yoakam, & Edwards, 2003) and mark a 10-year milestone in the community's journey to understand and meet the needs of its members. The earlier survey results informed development of a region-wide service provider readiness assessment, LGBT cultural competency training programming for service providers (Knochel, Quam, & Croghan, 2011) and plans for an LGBT welcoming senior housing project. This type of sequential survey work allows a community to assess change over time and determine the appropriate direction for future LGBT aging work. In this case, the 10-year follow-up survey revealed the LGBT community's persistent (a) lack of confidence that they would receive sensitive care if their sexual orientation or gender identity were know to the provider and (b) interest in seeking services from providers whose staff members had undergone training on LGBT aging issues. Both findings confirmed the community's commitment to continue to invest in the regional LGBT cultural competency training program.

Many of the reports included here obtained participants by recruiting through LGBT community organizations. Beyond recruiting research participants, this approach raises the profile of aging across the community, in circles that do not focus on older adults, perhaps even those that focus on youth. Research done in this manner serves as a reminder of the fact that the LGBT community is multifaceted and multigenerational with many needs and strengths.

CONCLUSION

Much of the community work contained in this special issue was necessary because questions about sexual orientation and gender identity are not regularly included in regional, state, and national planning research, nor in federal data sources. As policymakers and service providers consider allocation of scarce resources, locally generated datasets, such as these brought together in this special issue, document the characteristics of an often hidden community. They begin to build a profile of LGBT older adults, and provide data to encourage decision makers to support programs and services that will strengthen the LGBT aging experience.

REFERENCES

Adelman, M., Gurevitch, J., de Vries, B., & Blando, J. (2006). Openhouse: Community building and research in the LGBT aging population. In D. Kimmel, T. Rose, & S. David (Eds.), *Lesbian, gay, bisexual, and transgender aging: Research and clinical perspectives* (pp. 247–264). New York, NY: Columbia University Press.

American Psychiatric Association. (1973). *Homosexuality and sexual orientation disturbance: Proposed change in DSM II*. APA Document reference number 730008. Los Angeles, CA: American Psychiatric Association. Retrieved from http://www.torahdec.org/Downloads/DSM-II_Homosexuality_Revision.pdf

Badgett, L. (2002). *The myth of gay affluence and other tale tales: The political economy of sexual orientation*. San Diego, CA: University of California.

Balsam, K. F., Rothblum, E. D., & Beauchaine, T. P. (2005). Victimization over the life span: A comparison of lesbian, gay, bisexual, and heterosexual siblings. *Journal of Consulting & Clinical Psychology, 73*, 477–487.

Barker, J. C. (2002). Neighbors, friends and other nonkin caregivers of community-living dependent elders. *Journal of Gerontology: Social Sciences, 57*, 158–167.

Cantor, M. H., & Mayer, M. (1978). Factors in differential utilization of services by urban elderly. *Journal of Gerontological Social Work, 1*(1), 47–61.

Chin-Hong, P. V., Vittinghoff, V., Cranston, R. D., Buchbinder, S., Cohen, D., Colfax, G., Palefsky, J. M. (2004). Age-specific prevalence of anal human papillomavirus infection in HIV-negative sexually active men who have sex with men: The EXPLORE study. *Journal of Infectious Diseases, 190*, 2070–2076.

Croghan, C. (2011). *What works in the workplace: Thoughts on CCT*. Retrieved from http://www.asaging.org/blog/assessing-interest-lgbt-cultural-competency-training

Croghan, C., Mertens, A., Yoakam, J., & Edwards, N. (2003, April). *GLBT senior needs assessment*. Poster presented at the Aging in America conference, Chicago, IL.

D'Augelli, A., & Grossman, A. (2001). Disclosure of sexual orientation, victimization, and mental health among lesbian, gay, and bisexual older adults. *Journal of Interpersonal Violence, 16*, 1008–1027.

de Vries, B. (2006). Home at the end of the rainbow: Supportive housing for LGBT elders. *Generations, 29*, 64–69.

de Vries, B., & Blando, J. (2004). The study of gay and lesbian lives: Lessons for social gerontology. In G. Herdt & B. de Vries (Eds.), *Gay and lesbian aging: Research and future directions* (pp. 3–28). New York, NY: Springer.

de Vries, B., & Herdt, G. (2011). Gay men and aging. In T. M. Witten & A. E. Eyler (Eds.), *Gay, lesbian, bisexual, and transgender aging: Challenges in research, practice, and policy* (pp. 84–129). Baltimore, MD: Johns Hopkins University Press.

de Vries, B., Mason, A., Quam, J., & Acquaviva, K. (2009). State recognition of same-sex relationships and preparations for end of life among lesbian and gay boomers. *Sexuality Research and Social Policy, 6*(1), 90–101.

de Vries, B., & Megathlin, D. (2009). The meaning of friends for gay men and lesbians in the second half of life. *Journal of GLBT Family Studies, 5*, 82–98.

Frazer, M. S. (2009). *LGBT health and human services needs in New York state*. Albany, NY: Empire State Pride Agenda Foundation. Retrieved from http://www.prideagenda.org/Portals/0/pdfs/LGBT%20Health%20and%20Hum an%20Services%20Needs%20in%20New%20York%20State.

Fredriksen-Goldsen, K. I., Kim, H.-J., Emlet, C. A., Muraco, A., Erosheva, E. A., Hoy-Ellis, C. P., . . . Petry, H. (2011). *Aging and health report: Disparities and resilience among lesbian, gay, bisexual, and transgender older adults*. Seattle, WA: Institute for Multigenerational Health.

Grossman, A. H., D'Augelli, A. R., & O'Connell, T. S. (2001). Being lesbian, gay, bisexual, and 60 or older in North America. *Journal of Gay & Lesbian Social Services: Issues in Practice, Policy, & Research, 13*(4), 23–40.

Gruskin, E. P., Greenwood, G. L., Matevia, M., Pollack, L. M., & Bye, L. L. (2007). Disparities in smoking between the lesbian, gay, and bisexual population and the general population in California. *American Journal of Public Health, 97*, 1496–1502.

Herdt, G., & Kertzner, R. (2006). I do, but I can't: The impact of marriage denial on the mental health and sexual citizenship of lesbians and gay men in the United States. *Sexuality Research and Social Policy, 3*(1), 33–49.

Herek, G. M. (2006). Legal recognition of same-sex relationships in the United States. *American Psychologist, 61*, 607–621.

Institute of Medicine. (2011). *The health of lesbian, gay, bisexual, and transgender people: Building a foundation for better understanding*. Washington, DC: National Academies Press.

Kimmel, D. C. (1978). Adult development and aging: A gay perspective. *Journal of Social Issues, 34*(3), 113–130.

Knochel, K. A., Quam, J. K., & Croghan, C. F. (2011). Are old lesbian and gay people well served? Understanding the perceptions, preparation, and experiences of aging service providers. *Journal of Applied Gerontology, 30*, 370–389.

Kochman, A. (1997). Gay and lesbian elderly: Historical overview and implications for social work practice. In J. Quam (Ed.), *Social services for senior gay men and lesbians* (pp. 1–25). New York, NY: Haworth.

Massachusetts Department of Public Health. (2009). *The health of lesbian, gay, bisexual and transgender (LGBT) persons in Massachusetts: A survey of health issues comparing LGBT persons with their heterosexual and non-transgender counterparts*. Boston, MA: Author.

Maupin, A. (2007). *Michael Tolliver lives*. San Francisco, CA: HarperCollins.

MetLife Mature Market Institute. (2010). *Still out, still aging*. Westport, CT: Author.

Meyer, I. H. (2003). Prejudice, social stress, and mental health in lesbian, gay, and bisexual populations: Conceptual issues and research evidence. *Psychological Bulletin, 129*, 674–697.

Mills, T. C., Paul, J., Stall, R., Pollack, L., Canchola, J., Chang, Y. J, Catania, J. A. (2004). Distress and depression in men who have sex with men: The Urban Men's Health Study. *American Journal of Psychiatry, 161*, 278–285.

Minnesota Board on Aging. (2005). *Survey of older Minnesotans*. St. Paul, MN: Minnesota Board on Aging.

Movement Advancement Project. (2010). *Improving the lives of LGBT older adults*. Retrieved from http://www.sageusa.org/uploads/Advancing%20Equality%20for%20LGBT%20Elders%20%5BFINAL%20COMPRESSED%5D.

National Senior Citizens Law Center. (2011). *LGBT older adults in long-term care facilities: Stories from the field*. Retrieved from http://www.lgbtagingcenter.org/resources/resource.cfm?r=54

Quam, J., & Croghan, C. (2008). Evolving words, evolving categories: A challenge for LGBT aging research. *OutWord, 14*(4), 1.

Radloff, L. S. (1977). The CES-D scale: A self report depression scale for research in the general population. *Applied Psychological Measurement, 1*(1), 385–401.

Rawls, T. (2001). Disclosure and depression among older gay and homosexual men: Findings from the Urban Men's Health Study. In G. Herdt & B. de Vries (Eds.), *Gay and lesbian aging: Research and future directions* (pp. 117–142). New York, NY: Springer.

Tang, H., Greenwood, G. L., Cowling, D. W., Lloyd, J. C., Roeseler, A. G., & Bal, D. G. (2004). Cigarette smoking among lesbians, gays, and bisexuals: How serious a problem? (United States). *Cancer Causes & Control, 15*, 797–803.

Unger, R. K. (2000). Outsiders inside: Positive marginality and social change. *Journal of Social Issues, 56*(1), 163–179.

Valanis, B. G., Bowen, D. J., Bassford, T., Whitlock, E., Charney, P., & Carter, R. A. (2000). Sexual orientation and health: Comparisons in the women's health initiative sample. *Archives of Family Medicine, 9*, 843–853.

Wallace, S. P., Cochran, S. D., Durazo, E. M., & Ford, C. L. (2011). *The health of aging lesbian, gay and bisexual adults in California*. Los Angeles, CA: UCLA Center for Health Policy Research.

Wight, R., LeBlanc, A., de Vries, B., & Detels, R. (2012). Stress and mental health among midlife and older gay-identified men. *American Journal of Public Health*, e1–e8.

Social Care Networks and Older LGBT Adults: Challenges for the Future

MARK BRENNAN-ING, PhD

AIDS Community Research Initiative of America (ACRIA), ACRIA Center on HIV & Aging,
New York, New York; New York University College of Nursing, New York, New York, USA

LIZ SEIDEL, MSW

AIDS Community Research Initiative of America (ACRIA), ACRIA Center on HIV & Aging,
New York, New York, USA

BRITTA LARSON, MNA

Center on Halsted, Chicago, Illinois, USA

STEPHEN E. KARPIAK, PhD

AIDS Community Research Initiative of America (ACRIA), ACRIA Center on HIV & Aging,
New York, New York, USA

Research on service needs among older adults rarely addresses the special circumstances of lesbian, gay, bisexual, and transgender (LGBT) individuals, such as their reliance on friend-centered social networks or the experience of discrimination from service providers. Limited data suggests that older LGBT adults underutilize health and social services that are important in maintaining independence and quality of life. This study explored the social care networks of this population using a mixed-methods approach. Data were obtained from 210 LGBT older adults. The average age was 60 years, and 71% were men, 24% were women, and 5% were transgender or intersex. One-third was Black, and 62% were Caucasian. Quantitative assessments found high levels of morbidity and friend-centered support networks. Need for and use of services

We thank Betty Akins, Hope Barrett, Philonise Keithley, and Zach Zimmerman for their assistance in conducting the field effort for the study in Chicago. We also thank Sheila Massinde for her help with data preparation, cleaning, and data entry. Last, but not least, we are truly grateful to the over 200 lesbian, gay, bisexual, and transgender older adults who took the time to share their lives with us.

was frequently reported. Content analysis revealed unmet needs for basic supports, including housing, economic supports, and help with entitlements. Limited opportunities for socialization were strongly expressed, particularly among older lesbians. Implications for senior programs and policies are discussed.

Although the National Institutes of Health and the National Institute on Aging have identified the need to reduce health disparities in disadvantaged and minority populations, a dearth of knowledge on issues affecting lesbian, gay, bisexual, and transgender (LGBT) adults, and especially older adults, persists (Fredriksen-Goldsen, Kim, Emlet, Muraco, & Erosheva, 2011; Knochel, Quam, & Croghan, 2011). Recognizing this need to include older LGBT adults has begun to be directly addressed by the federal government. The Department of Health and Human Services (HHS) has recently partnered with SAGE (Services and Advocacy for GLBT Elders) to create the National Resource Center on LGBT Aging (SAGE, 2013a). In addition, the U.S. HHS Secretary announced that the agency will integrate questions on sexual orientation into data collection efforts by 2013 (U.S. HHS, 2011), building on the recommendations of the Institute of Medicine (IOM; 2011) report. Thus, there is a growing consensus that additional research is needed on LGBT older adults to better meet the needs of this population.

SOCIAL CARE NEEDS OF OLDER LGBT ADULTS

Given our existing albeit limited knowledge of LGBT aging, one area of concern is their ability to access adequate social care in as they age. As defined by Cantor and Brennan (2000), social care includes the broad-based system of informal social network resources (i.e., family and friends) and the network of community-based formal services (e.g., senior centers, home health care). The social care network is considered to be a vital component of helping people to age independently and maintain quality of life, and is the focus of this article on older LGBT adults.

The dynamics of the social care network are illustrated by the *Hierarchical Compensatory Theory* of social supports (Cantor & Mayer, 1978). This theory posits that when older people need assistance, they turn first to close family members such as spouses or children. If these individuals are not available, they will then turn to more distant relatives, then friends and neighbors, and, finally, to formal community-based supports in a hierarchical manner. Formal services are increasingly accessed when informal caregivers are unable to meet the needs of the older adults (Cantor & Brennan, 2000). Support for the Hierarchical Compensatory Theory is evidenced in findings that older adults using formal services were more likely than their peers to live alone (i.e., not have a partner or spouse) and to be disadvantaged in health and economic resources (Cantor & Brennan, 1993). Other studies report that socially isolated older adults often use community-based supports, such as religious congregations for their needs, viewing them as "surrogate families" (Sheehan, Wilson, & Marella, 1988; Tirrito & Choi, 2005).

Research suggests that the LGBT population may have different health needs when compared with their heterosexual counterparts. Such differences can affect the social care needs of this population. For example, LGBT individuals report poorer health than the general population (Wallace, Cochran, Durazo, & Ford, 2011). Higher disability rates have also been reported, with one study reporting 47% of older LGBT adults having at least one disability (Fredriksen-Goldsen et al., 2011; Wallace et al., 2011). HIV infection is also a dominant health issue within the LGBT community. Data from the Centers for Disease Control and Prevention (CDC; 2010) show that 55% of all new HIV infections occur among men who have sex with men, and 17% occur among people age 50 and older. As a result of effective antiretroviral treatments, it is estimated that the majority of people living with HIV will be 50 and older by 2015 (Effros et al., 2008). Significantly, older adults with HIV are evidencing the early onset of age-related illnesses, such as cardiovascular disease and osteoporosis, that are typically associated with the very old (Havlik, Brennan, & Karpiak, 2011).

Older lesbians have higher rates of obesity compared to heterosexual women, which negatively affects their health by increasing the risk for condition such as diabetes, cardiac disease, and certain cancers (Fredriksen-Goldsen et al., 2011; IOM, 2011). The problem of obesity among African American lesbians is worse, and this condition is exacerbated among those who live in either urban or rural areas, and are of lower socioeconomic status (Substance Abuse and Mental Health Services Administration [SAMSA], 2012). Lower rates of pregnancy and underutilization of PAP smears and mammograms puts lesbians at higher risk for reproductive cancers (U.S. HHS, 2010; SAMSA, 2012). Care for lesbian and bisexual women is often compromised because they are reluctant to disclose their sexual identities to health care providers, fearing poor treatment or negative reactions (Stein & Bonuck, 2001).

According to the American Lung Association (2010), tobacco smokers are at greatest risk for lung cancer, and gay and bisexual men are more likely to smoke than their peers in the general population. Lesbians are more likely to smoke than heterosexual women. Among older LGBT adults, one study found a 50% lifetime smoking rate with 10% currently smoking (Fredriksen-Goldsen et al., 2011). Smoking tobacco accounts for the vast majority of lung cancers (87%) and is linked to other serious conditions such as heart disease, stroke, and emphysema. Those living with HIV may be at further risk as research finds that HIV makes the lungs less able to recover from smoking damage. Given that smoking is commonplace in bars and clubs that are frequent social venues for older LGBT adults, exposure to secondhand smoke may also increase health risks in this population (American Lung Association, 2010).

Poor mental health has been identified as an issue in LGBT populations (IOM, 2011) and is also linked to poorer health outcomes (Havlik et al., 2011). Fredriksen-Goldsen et al. (2011) found that one-third of their participants met the clinical threshold for depression. In addition nearly 10% of older LGBT adults in this study used alcohol excessively and consumed drugs that were not prescribed to them. These high rates of morbidity and prevalence of mental health and substance use issues suggest that many LGBT adults will face health challenges as they age and will require assistance from their social care networks to maintain independence and a decent quality of life in the coming decades.

THE INFORMAL SOCIAL NETWORKS OF OLDER LGBT ADULTS

As aging LGBT adults increasingly require social care, their informal social networks are a cause for concern. Research finds that LGBT older adults typically do not have the robust informal social resources that characterize those from heterosexual communities. Among heterosexual older adults, it is the spouse and children who are the most likely to provide needed assistance and support (Cantor & Brennan, 2000). Among community-dwelling older adults, 43% report a spouse, whereas 77% have at least one living child (Cantor & Brennan, 1993). However, among older LGBT adults, approximately 40% have a partner or spouse, and only 20% to 25% report at least one living child (Cantor, Brennan, & Shippy, 2004; Fredriksen-Goldsen et al., 2011). Thus, the social networks of older LGBT adults are characterized by reliance on the "family of choice" comprising close friends and neighbors, in contrast to the biological family or "family of origin" that is the foundation for most heterosexual older adults (de Vries & Hoctel, 2007; Dorfman, Walters, Burke, Hardin, & Karanik, 1995; Grossman, D'Augelli, & Hershberger, 2000; Shippy, Cantor, & Brennan, 2004).

While the importance of friends in the lives of LGBT older adults is well documented, there may be limits in their ability to provide care to them over the long term, especially if decision making is required (Fredriksen-Goldsen et al., 2011). The absence of blood ties between friends who comprise the family of choice and the older LGBT adult can result in negative interactions with the biological family. In addition, the lack of legal recognition of same-sex partners in most jurisdictions excludes these individuals from making caregiving decisions concerning their significant others (Cantor et al., 2004).

SERVICE UTILIZATION BY LGBT OLDER ADULTS

Given the limited social networks of older LGBT adults, many will need to rely on formal community-based supports to meet their needs as they grow older. LGBT adults, including older adults, face barriers when accessing care including assumption of heterosexuality, lack of same-sex partner recognition, and disparate treatment by providers manifested by discrimination springing from negative attitudes toward the LGBT population (Brotman, Ryan, & Cormier, 2003; Cantor et al., 2004; M. Hughes, 2007; Tan, 2005). Tjepkema (2008) found that such barriers result in reduced access to services and increased unmet needs. An IOM (2011) report concluded that LGBT adults face barriers due to a lack of culturally competent providers and fear of discrimination, both of which promote health disparities in this population. Fredriksen-Goldsen et al. (2011) found that over 10% of LGBT older adults reported receiving sub-par care or being denied care. Clover (2006), in a qualitative study of gay men between the ages of 60 and 70, found many hesitated to receive aging services because they anticipated being discriminated against and not receiving optimal care. Overt discrimination aside, research shows that many mental health, substance use, aging and health services organizations do not have enough information or training about LGBT individuals to serve them in a culturally competent manner (A. K. Hughes, Harold, & Boyer, 2011; Israel, Walther, Gortcheva, & Perry, 2011; Knochel et al., 2011).

PURPOSE AND RATIONALE

LGBT older adults face numerous challenges as they age, including high levels of physical and mental health morbidity, limited social networks that may be not be able to meet their needs, and continued barriers to service such as discrimination, heterosexist attitudes, and a lack of cultural competence on the part of providers. Many of these older adults will have a greater need to access formal community-based supports as they grow older. In 2010, the older adult program at the Center on Halsted (COH) in Chicago was awarded a generous grant from the Human Resources Services Administration to enhance the live of LGBT older adults. COH recognized that there was a dearth of research addressing the needs of older adults that would be useful for policy, advocacy and program planning, and set aside a significant portion of these funds to conduct a comprehensive study of the health and psychosocial needs of older LGBT adults in Chicago. Drawing from these data, the purpose of this article is to examine the social care network of older LGBT adults, with a focus on the viability of the social support network, formal service utilization, and unmet needs for assistance. After providing a demographic and health profile of a sample of these older LGBT adults, we then describe their informal social networks, service utilization patterns, and services needs based on quantitative measures. This is followed by a qualitative examination of unmet service needs that provides more comprehensive insight of the issues faced by these older adults as they access social care resources.

METHOD

Samples and Procedures

Data were obtained in 2010 and 2011 from a convenience sample of older LGBT adults recruited through the COH, the most comprehensive LGBT community center in the Midwest. COH offers diverse public programs and social services, including mental health counseling, HIV testing and prevention, community and cultural programs, technology classes, youth programs, and a vibrant older adult program for those 55 and older. Participants were also recruited at and at various AIDS service organizations (ASOs), health fairs, and community events in Chicago, IL. To qualify for participation an individual had to identify as LGBT and be 50 years of age or older and sufficiently fluent in English to complete the survey. Two hundred thirty-three participants were recruited resulting in 210 usable surveys. Twenty-three surveys were not usable due to incomplete data or from participants who failed to meet the inclusion criteria (most often for not being LGBT). Informed consent was obtained prior to data collection. The survey instrument was self-administered and took, on average, 45 to 60 min to complete. After completion participants were debriefed, thanked, and given a $25 gift card. Research methods and materials were evaluated and approved by the Copernicus Group Independent Review Board.

Quantitative Measures

Whenever possible standardized measures with known psychometric properties were used to insure validity and allow for comparison with published data. Questions were developed based on items in Research on Older Adults with HIV study (Brennan et al., 2009), National Social Life, Health and Aging Project (Lindau et al., 2007), and the Caregiving among Older Lesbian, Gay, Bisexual and Transgender New Yorkers study (Cantor et al., 2004).

Demographic profile. Single items obtained information on *age, gender identity* (i.e., male, female, male-to-female transgender, female-to-male transgender, or intersex), *sexual identity* (i.e., heterosexual, homosexual, bisexual, queer, or questioning), *race, Hispanic origin, level of education, income adequacy, work status, HIV status, veteran's status,* and *marital or partnership status* (see Table 1).

TABLE 1 Sociodemographic Characteristics of Older Lesbian, Gay, Bisexual, and Transgender Adults (Valid Percentages)

Variable	Total		Men		Women	
	n	%	*n*	%	*n*	%
Age						
M	59.6		59.9		58.4	
SD	8.00		8.41		6.57	
Age group						
50–54	67	32.4	48	32.7	17	35.4
55–59	51	24.6	32	21.8	13	27.1
60–64	34	16.4	27	18.4	7	14.6
65–69	30	14.5	19	12.9	9	18.8
70+	25	12.1	21	14.3	2	4.2
Gender						
Male	148	70.5	148	100.0		
Female	50	23.7			50	23.7
Transgender male	1	0.5				
Transgender female	10	4.8				
Intersex	1	0.5				
Sexual identity						
Gay/lesbian	165	80.1	116	80.0	44	88.0
Bisexual	28	13.6	23	15.9	3	6.0
Queer	7	3.4	5	3.4	1	2.0
Questioning	3	1.5	1	0.7	2	4.0
Heterosexual	3	1.5				
Race/ethnicity						
Black/African American	66	32.0	47	32.0	14	29.8
White/Caucasian	127	61.7	92	62.6	30	63.8
Hispanic	8	3.9	6	4.1	2	4.3
Asian/Pacific Islander	1	0.5	1	0.7	0	0.0
American Indian/Alaskan Native	1	0.5	0	0.0	1	2.1
Other	3	1.5	1	0.7	0	0.0
Education						
Less than high school	10	4.9	6	4.2	2	4.1
High school graduate/GED	31	15.2	24	16.7	4	8.2
Some college	50	24.5	33	22.9	12	24.5
College graduate/postgraduate	113	55.4	81	56.2	31	63.3
Income adequacy						
Not enough for expenses	32	15.5	23	15.9	6	12.0
Just manage to get by	94	45.6	68	46.9	20	40.0
Enough with a little extra	46	22.3	31	21.4	14	28.0
Money not a problem	34	16.5	23	15.9	10	20.0

(Continued)

TABLE 1 (Continued)

Variable	Total		Men		Women	
	n	%	*n*	%	*n*	%
Work status**						
Working	58	27.9	32	21.9	25	50.0
Unemployed	26	12.5	21	14.4	4	8.0
Disability	62	29.8	46	31.5	9	18.0
Retired	58	27.9	45	30.8	10	20.0
Volunteer	2	1.0	1	0.7	1	2.0
Other	2	1.0	1	0.7	1	2.0
Military veteran**	28	13.4	26	17.6	1	2.0
Marital/partnership status*						
Married	8	3.9	5	3.5	2	4.1
Civil union	2	1.0	2	1.4	0	0.0
Registered domestic partner	10	4.9	3	2.1	7	14.3
Life partner	50	24.4	35	24.3	15	30.6
Common law	1	0.5	0	0.0	0	0.0
Widowed/partner deceased	8	3.9	8	5.6	0	0.0
Divorced/separated	19	9.3	12	8.3	4	8.2
Single/not married	107	52.2	79	54.9	21	42.9

Note. $N = 210$ (men, $n = 148$; women, $n = 50$). GED = general equivalency diploma.
*$p < .05$. **$p < .01$.

Morbidity. Participants were asked if they had experienced any of 27 physical and mental health conditions in the previous year, including HIV-related conditions (e.g., neuropathy), age-related conditions (e.g., sensory loss), chronic and terminal illnesses (e.g., diabetes or cancer), and mental or neurological disorders (e.g., depression). The number of health comorbidities was calculated by summing the positive responses to these items.

Self-rated health. Participants rated their current health status on a 4-point Likert scale (i.e., from *excellent* to *poor*).

Depression. The 10-item version of the Center for Epidemiological Studies Depression Scale (CES–D; Radloff, 1977) was used to assess depressive symptoms (Andersen, Malmgren, Carter, & Patrick, 1994). Participants were asked about the frequency of depressive symptoms experienced over the past week, with four responses (i.e., none, a little, some, or most days). Responses were summed with higher scores indicating greater levels of depressive symptoms. Inter-item reliability for the CES–D was high (Cronbach's = .84). CES–D scores were then categorized (i.e., not depressed = 0 to 9, moderately depressed = 10 to 13, or severe depression = 14 to 30; Andersen et al., 1994).

Functional ability was measured using the Older Americans Resources and Services assessment (Fillenbaum, 1988). Respondents were asked about any difficulty they encountered with seven instrumental activities of daily living (IADLs) and six personal care activities of daily living (PADLs), with

TABLE 2 Physical and Mental Health Status of Older Lesbian, Gay, Bisexual, and Transgender Adults (Valid Percentages)

	Total		Men		Women	
Variable	M	SD	M	SD	M	SD
Number of health conditions	2.98	2.42	3.05	2.47	2.33	1.91
CES–D	8.25	5.89	8.04	6.16	8.42	5.19
Number of difficult IADLs	0.98	1.57	1.01	1.62	0.80	1.44
Number of difficult PADLs	0.41	1.15	0.39	1.10	0.42	1.31
	n	%	n	%	n	%
Self-rated health						
Excellent	57	27.1	43	29.5	11	22.0
Good	100	47.6	73	50.0	23	46.0
Fair	43	20.5	28	19.2	12	24.0
Poor	8	3.8	2	1.4	4	8.0
CES–D categories**						
Not depressed	135	64.3	101	68.2	28	56.0
Moderately depressed	33	15.7	15	10.1	15	30.0
Severely depressed	42	20.0	32	21.6	7	14.0
At least 1 IADL impairment	78	37.1	56	37.8	16	32.0
At least 1 ADL impairment	36	17.1	24	16.2	7	14.0
Insurance and benefits[a]						
Medicare*	93	44.7	72	48.6	16	32.0
Medicaid	56	26.9	39	26.4	9	18.0
Private health insurance*	88	42.3	59	39.9	29	58.0
Long-term care insurance	19	9.1	13	8.8	6	12.0
VA health coverage	14	6.7	13	8.8	1	2.0
Private disability policy	6	2.9	4	2.7	2	4.0
Supplemental security income	45	21.6	31	20.9	8	16.0
Social Security Disability Income	44	21.2	34	14.0	7	20.7
General assistance	5	2.4	5	3.4	0	0.0
Supplemental nutrition Assistance program	54	26.0	37	25.0	10	20.0

Note. N = 210 (men, n = 148; women, n = 50). CES–D = Center for Epidemiological Studies Depression Scale; IADLs = instrumental activities of daily living; PADLs = personal care activities of daily living; VA = Veterans' Administration.

[a]Multiple response categories. Totals do not equal 100%.

*p < .05. **p < .01.

higher scores indicating more difficulty. For these analyses, the number of activities with any difficulty reported was summed in both IADL and PADL domains. The proportion of respondents with at least one impairment in each domain was also calculated (see Table 2).

Insurance and benefits were assessed by asking about government health insurance (e.g., Medicaid), private insurance, long-term care and disability coverage, and various entitlement programs (e.g., Supplemental Security Income [SSI]; see Table 2).

Living arrangement was assessed by asking respondents if they lived alone or with others, and if living with others, the nature of that relationship.

Informal social network. Detailed information was collected on informal networks based on previous large-scale studies of older adults (Cantor & Brennan, 1993, 2000). Participants indicate if they have any living members of five groups (e.g., parents, children, sibling, other relatives, and friends) that typically compromise informal networks, and the number of those network elements present. Two additional items assessed frequency of contact (e.g., in-person visits or telephone conversations). Assessments of contact frequency was necessary to calculate the functional status of each network element, based on criteria established by Cantor (Cantor, 1979)—namely, monthly in-person visits or weekly telephone conversations. The proportion of respondents having at least one functional network element in each of the five categories was then calculated. Respondents were also asked the number of neighbors known well and the number of their friends who had HIV/AIDS.

Type and frequency of assistance from family and friends. Participants indicated the frequency of eight types of instrumental and emotional assistance provided by family members and friends, respectively (e.g., shop or run errands, help with housekeeping, advice, and talk about personal problems). Respondents were also asked about negative support received from either family or friends (e.g., upset you or hurt your feelings). These responses were summed to create indexes of family/friend help and negative support (see Table 3).

Formal service utilization. Questions on services accessed in the previous year in addition to those received at the COH were adapted from previous studies of service utilization among older adults (Cantor & Brennan, 1993, 2000). The time frame of the previous year was retained so as to facilitate comparisons between the study sample and other data. Four categories were assessed: (a) government agencies and offices (e.g., Medicaid), (b) HIV/AIDS-related services (e.g., HIV day program), (c) health and long-term care services (e.g., emergency room), and (d) other older adult services (e.g., senior center). The number of services used within each of the four categories and overall was summed to create variables indicating the total number of services used the number used in each domain (see Table 4).

Service needs in the previous year. Respondents were asked about 11 service needs in the previous year in four domains: *socialization* (e.g., someone to call or visit), *social services* (e.g., help with entitlements), *household tasks* (e.g., home repairs), and *health-related* (e.g., care after a hospital stay). Positive responses to these items were summed to create an index of service needs in the previous year (see Table 5).

Open-ended questions on service needs. The narrative data used for the qualitative examination of service needs in the previous year was taken from two questions. The first item asked, "We are interested in knowing more about why people did not get all the help they needed. If you did not receive all of the help you needed, please tell us in your own words about

TABLE 3 Social Network Characteristics (Valid Percentages)

Variable	Total		Men		Women	
	n	%	*n*	%	*n*	%
Living arrangements***						
Live alone	131	63.3	105	70.5	18	39.1
Live with spouse or partner	44	21.3	25	16.8	18	39.1
Live with other	32	15.5	19	12.8	10	21.7
Social network members						
Parent	86	41.7	65	44.5	18	36.7
Functional parent	55	26.1	41	27.5	13	26.0
Child**	64	30.9	36	24.5	23	47.9
Functional child***	48	22.7	23	15.4	21	42.0
Grandchild*	43	20.8	25	17.2	16	32.0
Functional grandchild**	20	9.5	9	6.0	10	20.0
Sibling	174	84.1	121	82.9	44	88.0
Functional sibling*	81	38.4	53	35.6	27	54.0
Other relative in contact	100	50.3	72	50.7	25	54.3
Friend	179	86.1	127	86.4	43	86.0
Functional friend	162	76.8	114	76.5	39	78.0
	M	*SD*	*M*	*SD*	*M*	*SD*
No. of friends with HIV**	0.81	1.63	1.05	1.84	0.18	0.51
No. of neighbors known well	1.49	2.80	1.42	2.66	1.60	2.10
Size of social network**	10.58	7.37	9.87	6.80	12.98	8.51
No. of ways family helps**	1.94	2.05	1.72	1.92	2.64	2.15
No. of ways friends help	2.20	2.06	2.06	1.96	2.40	2.05
Family negative support**	0.68	0.99	0.54	0.90	1.02	1.07
Friend negative support	0.46	0.87	0.46	0.80	0.44	1.01

Note. $N = 210$ (men, $n = 148$; women, $n = 50$).
$*p < .05. **p < .01. ***p < .001.$

the situation." The second question asked, "Are there any other programs or services that could be helpful to you from Center on Halsted or other service providers?"

Design and Analysis

This study used a mixed methods approach incorporating both quantitative and qualitative data analyses. The quantitative portion used a correlational design to assess how demographic factors, health status, informal network characteristics, formal service utilization, and service needs were associated with gender. Due to the small number of transgender and intersex respondents (i.e., $n = 12$; see Table 1), it was not possible to include these individuals in significance testing by gender identity, but they were included in reporting the total descriptive information for the sample reported in Tables 1 through 5. Differences in study variables by gender identity were assessed using chi-square analyses for nominal and ordinal data and analyses of variance for continuous data. When noted in the text, "significant" refers to statistically significant differences at the $p < .05$ level or greater. For the

TABLE 4 Services Used by Older Lesbian, Gay, Bisexual, and Transgender Adults in the Past Year (Valid Percentages)

Variable	Total		Men		Women	
	n	%	*n*	%	*n*	%
Government offices/agencies						
Social Security office	90	42.7	65	43.6	17	34.0
Medicare office	43	20.5	33	22.3	7	14.0
Medicaid office	42	19.9	28	18.8	8	16.0
VA hospital	16	7.6	14	9.4	2	4.0
HRA	42	20.0	32	21.6	5	10.0
Chicago Housing Authority	43	20.5	32	21.6	6	12.0
Police	25	11.9	15	10.1	8	16.0
Department on Aging	57	27.1	41	27.7	10	20.0
ASOs						
AIDS Foundation of Chicago***	43	26.2	40	33.1	1	3.1
BEHIV*	18	11.0	18	15.0	0	0.0
COH HIV services	49	30.2	39	32.5	7	21.9
Chicago House and Social Services	20	12.3	18	15.0	2	6.2
Howard Brown Health Services	41	25.5	34	28.6	5	15.6
Test Positive Aware Network**	30	18.4	29	24.2	0	0.0
South Side Help Center	11	6.7	9	7.5	2	6.2
CORE Center*	21	13.0	19	16.0	1	3.1
Chicago Women's AIDS Project	9	5.6	8	6.7	0	0.0
Health and LTC						
Private medical clinic	68	33.0	46	31.5	21	42.9
Health maintenance organization	23	11.1	18	12.2	4	8.2
Dentist/dental clinic	101	48.8	68	46.6	30	60.0
Mental health services	56	27.2	36	24.7	15	30.6
Drug/alcohol treatment	23	11.3	19	13.2	4	8.2
Emergency room	56	27.1	37	25.2	17	34.7
Inpatient hospital	39	18.9	25	17.1	12	24.5
Outpatient hospital	77	37.6	56	38.6	20	40.8
Case management*	59	28.5	48	32.7	8	16.3
Homecare services	36	17.4	24	16.3	8	16.3
Assisted living	10	4.8	5	3.4	5	10.2
Hospice	6	3.0	3	2.1	1	2.1
CBOs						
Senior center	52	25.2	32	21.9	14	28.6
Meal/nutrition program	41	19.8	27	18.4	10	20.4
Self-help group	30	14.5	22	15.0	6	12.2
Clergy**	47	22.7	40	27.2	4	8.2
Legal services	43	20.8	31	21.1	9	18.4
COH senior services						
Mental health support	21	10.5	15	10.5	3	6.5
HIV support group**	20	10.3	20	14.4	0	0.0
Congregate meals	69	35.6	48	34.8	14	31.1
Legal assistance*	21	10.8	18	12.9	1	2.3
Computer technology center	52	26.4	38	27.1	8	17.4
Social/education programs	54	27.8	34	24.8	15	31.9

(Continued)

TABLE 4 (Continued)

	M	SD	M	SD	M	SD
Government services used	1.70	1.95	1.75	1.95	1.26	1.76
ASOs used***	1.20	1.79	1.50	1.93	0.36	0.78
Health/LTC services used	2.63	2.27	2.58	2.19	2.90	2.54
CBOs used	1.01	1.18	1.02	1.16	0.86	1.23
COH services	1.12	1.29	1.16	1.25	0.82	1.26
Total no. of services[a]	6.48	5.14	6.85	5.19	5.38	4.94

Note. N = 210 (men, *n* = 148; women, *n* = 50). VA = Veterans' Administration; HRA = Human Resources Administration; ASOs = AIDS service organizations; COH = Center on Halsted; BEHIV = Better Existence with HIV; LTC = long-term care; CBOs = community-based organizations.
[a]Does not include Center on Halsted Services due to overlap with other items.
*$p < .05$. **$p < .01$. ***$p < .001$.

TABLE 5 Need for Services in the Past Year Among Older Lesbian, Gay, Bisexual, and Transgender Adults (Valid Percentages)

	Total		Men		Women	
Variable	*n*	%	*n*	%	*n*	%
Number services needed						
M	2.48		2.44		2.54	
SD	2.25		2.26		2.23	
Socialization						
Someplace to socialize	105	51.0	76	52.1	23	47.9
Someone to call or visit	52	25.4	35	23.8	13	27.7
Social Services						
Personal/family counseling	59	28.6	40	27.4	14	29.2
Help with entitlements*	47	22.7	39	26.7	6	12.2
Finding a job*	37	18.0	31	21.2	4	8.3
Household						
Home repairs**	45	23.0	28	18.9	17	35.4
Housekeeping/personal care	37	18.2	22	15.5	12	24.5
Home-delivered meals	8	3.8	4	2.7	4	8.2
Health-related						
Escort to doctor or clinic	65	31.6	41	27.7	19	39.6
Care after hospital stay	42	20.5	29	20.1	10	20.4
Visiting nurse/home health care	25	12.3	18	12.3	5	10.6

Note. N = 210 (men, *n* = 148; women, *n* = 50).
*$p < .05$. **$p < .01$.

sake of brevity, only significant differences based on gender are described in the results.

The qualitative portion of the study used a grounded-theory approach (Glaser & Strauss, 1967)—namely, codes and themes were not identified *a priori,* but were developed through a process of open coding. Narrative data from the two open-ended questions were imported into the qualitative analysis program *ATLAS.ti* (Muhr, 1997). Mark Brennan-Ing conducted the open-coding process in an iterative process by identifying content and themes and corresponding coding, refining the coding system by making several passes through the data using the method of constant comparisons. Following this phase, Liz Seidel independently reviewed the initial coding and themes and noted any disagreement both with regard to the passages that were coded, as well as the codes themselves. The proportion of agreements and disagreements between Mark Brennan-Ing and Liz Seidel were calculated and disagreements were resolved through discussion. Interrater agreement for the open-coding phase was 94%. Because the interrater agreement for the open-coding phase was very high, a focused coding phase was not deemed necessary and the initial coding was corrected to reflect the consensus of Mark Brennan-Ing and Liz Seidel.

RESULTS

Sociodemographic and Socioeconomic Characteristics

The average age of this sample of older LGBT adults was 59.5 years, and ranged from 50 to 92 years of age. The median age was 58 years. The majority identified as male (71%), with 24% identifying as female, and 5% as transgender female. One individual identified as a transgender male (0.5%) and one identified as intersex (0.5%). Due to the small numbers of transgender and intersex individuals, they were not included in the bivariate comparisons by gender of the quantitative data that follow, but were included in the qualitative analysis of service needs (see Table 1). Eighty percent identified as gay or lesbian, 14% as bisexual, 1% as queer, and 3 transgender individuals (1%) identified as heterosexual. The majority of the sample was White (62%), followed by Black (32%). The remaining race/ethnicities ranged from 4.0% (Hispanic) to 0.5% (Asian/Pacific Islander and American Indian/Alaskan Native).

Educational attainment in this sample was high, with 55% having graduated from college or attended graduate school. Twenty-five percent had attended some college but not received a degree, and 15% had obtained a high school diploma or general equivalency diploma. Only 5% had less than high school educations. However, over one-half reported income inadequacy of either not having enough money for expenses (16%) or just managing to get by financially (46%). Nearly one-fourth said that they had enough money with a bit extra (22%), whereas 17% indicated that money was not a problem (see Table 1). With regard to current work status, comparable proportions were either working full time (28%), were retired (28%), or were disabled (30%). Twelve percent reported being unemployed. Work status differed significantly by gender with older women being significantly more likely than men to be working (50% vs. 22%), and less likely to report being retired (20% vs. 31%) or on disability (18% vs. 32%). The higher likelihood of disability among older men compared to lesbian and bisexual women is likely a reflection of the much higher prevalence of HIV in the former group compared with the latter (46% vs. 2%; $p < .001$). Thirteen percent reported having served in the military (see Table 1), and older gay and bisexual men were significantly more likely to be veterans as compared to lesbian and bisexual women (18% and 2%, respectively).

In terms of current marital/partnership status, 52% reported being single. The next largest group (35%) was those with a partner or spouse (life partners 24%, registered domestic partners 5%, married 4%, civil unions 1%, and common law 1%). Nine percent were divorced or separated and 4% reported being widowed or that their partner was deceased. Older lesbian and bisexual women were much more likely to say they had a partner (31% life partner and 14% domestic partner) as compared to their male peers (24% life partner and 2% domestic partner; see Table 1).

Health, Health Care, and Insurance

Physical and mental health. Respondents were asked if they had experienced any of 27 health conditions in the previous year, including age-related conditions (e.g., arthritis, cardiac conditions, cancer, depression, hepatitis, and HIV). As seen in Table 2, on average, older LGBT adults reported having three health conditions, and this did not differ significantly by gender. Despite this level of comorbidity, three-fourths self-rated their health as either excellent (27%) or good (48%). Twenty-one percent responded that they were in fair health, and only 4% rated their health as poor. The number of health conditions and self-rated health were not significantly related to gender.

Data on depressive symptomatology showed the study group had an average CES–D score of 8.3. Using the classification system developed by Andersen et al. (1994), 16% reported moderate levels of depressive symptoms, whereas one out of five had severe levels of depressive symptoms. Average CES–D scores did not differ significantly by gender. However, in terms of severity of symptoms, older gay and bisexual men were significantly more likely to have severe symptoms (22%) and less likely to have moderate symptoms (10%) as compared with older lesbian and bisexual women (14% and 30%, respectively; see Table 2).

Regarding functional ability, the IADL task with the most frequent reported difficulty was housework (25%). Difficulty getting to places out of walking distance (21%) and shopping (18%) were the next most difficult IADL, whereas 16% reported difficulty with meal preparation. Less than one 1 of 10 reported difficulty with using the telephone (5%), taking medications (5%) or handling money (8%). Thirty-seven percent reported difficulty with at least one IADL task (see Table 2), and reported 1.0 difficult IADL tasks, on average. Older LGBT adults were less likely to report difficulties with PADLs as compared with IADLs. The greatest reported difficulty was for getting in and out of bed (12%) and dressing/undressing (9%). Seven percent or less reported difficulty with the remaining PADLs; walking across a small room (7%), bathing (6%), grooming (5%), and feeding oneself (3%). Seventeen percent reported difficulty with at least one PADL task, and the average number of PADL difficulties was 0.4.

Health insurance and entitlement benefits. Medicare was the most frequently reported health insurance program (45%). Men were significantly more likely than women to report Medicare coverage (49% and 32%, respectively). This was followed by private health insurance (42%); however, women were more likely than men to report such coverage (58% and 40%, respectively). Slightly more than one-fourth of the sample was on Medicaid (27%), whereas relatively few reported long-term care insurance (9%), coverage through the Veterans' Administration (VA; 7%), or a private disability policy (3%). With regard to entitlements, about one-fifth reported either SSI or Social Security Disability Income (SSDI; see Table 2). Twenty-six percent reported being enrolled in the Supplemental Nutrition Program. Less than 2% were receiving welfare in the form of general assistance.

Social Network Composition and Social Support

Nearly two-thirds of the sample lived alone (63%), whereas 21% lived with a partner or spouse, and 16% lived with some other person (see Table 3). Men were significantly more likely to live alone compared to women (71% and 39%, respectively), and concomitantly less likely to live with a partner or spouse (17% and 39%, respectively). With regard to social network elements and functional elements, 42% reported the presence of a living parent. However, the proportion having a functional parent declined to 26%. (Note that a functional network member is in at least monthly face-to-face or weekly telephone contact.) Less than one-third (31%) reported the presence of a living child, whereas 23% reported having at least one functional child. Older gay and bisexual men were significantly less likely than their female counterparts to report a living child (25% and 48%, respectively). A similar picture emerged regarding functional children with women more likely than men to report a functional child (42% and 15%, respectively). Given their greater likelihood of having children, it was not surprising that women were significantly more likely to report both living grandchildren (32%) and functional grandchildren (20%) as compared with men (17% and 6%, respectively). Eighty-four percent reported a living sibling, but less than one-half of these could be categorized as functional (38%). One-half of the sample reported having other, more distant relative with whom they are in frequent contact.

The well-documented friend-centered nature of LGBT social networks, or so-called families of choice, was evident among the older adults in our sample. Eighty-six percent reported having a close friend, and 77% reported having a functional friend (see Table 3). On average, older LGBT adults reported 4.1 friends in their social networks, and approximately one out of four was HIV-positive ($M = 0.80$). Older gay and bisexual men had a significantly higher average number of friends with HIV as compared with women ($M = 1.05$ and $M = 0.18$, respectively). An additional source of non-kin support is from neighbors. Respondents reported knowing 1.5 neighbors well, on average (see Table 3). Older LGBT adults reported a mean of 10.6 individuals in their social networks. Women had significantly larger networks, on average ($M = 13$), as compared with men ($M = 10$). The larger size of social networks among women is due to their greater likelihood of having both children and grandchildren compared to men.

Support assistance and negative support. We asked older LGBT adults about the amount of assistance they received from family and friends in terms of instrumental help (i.e., shop/run errands, keep house/prepare meals, someone to take them to the doctor/clinic, help with mail/correspondence, and managing money) and emotional support (i.e., advice, need cheering up, and talk about personal matters). Respondents reported receiving 1.9 types of help, on average, from family. Women reported significantly greater help from family as compared to men ($M = 2.6$ and $M = 1.7$, respectively). With regard to help from friends, older LGBT adults reported 2.2 types of help from their families of choice, on average, and this did not differ significantly by gender. More important, the amount of support from friends was not significantly lower than that received from family, $t(210) = -1.63$, $p = .10$, underscoring the crucial role of non-kin support among older LGBT adults.

We also assessed negative social support from family and friends in terms of refusing to help when asked, being reluctant to talk, or upsetting/hurting the feelings of the respondent. On average, respondents reported 0.7 types of negative support from family. While older lesbian and bisexual women have larger family networks who provide greater levels of assistance, they are also significantly more likely than men to report higher levels of negative family support ($M = 1.0$ and $M = 0.5$, respectively). Respondents reported 0.5 types of negative support from friends, on average, and this was significantly less than negative support received from family, $t(210) = 2.89$, $p < .005$.

Service Utilization in the Previous Year

Government offices and agencies. The most frequently utilized service in this group was the Social Security Office (43%), followed by the Department for Family and Support Services, Senior Division/Department on Aging (27%). Next were the Chicago Housing Authority (21%) and Medicare and Medicaid Offices (21% and 20%, respectively). Twenty percent had also used the Department of Human Resources Administration in the previous year (see Table 4). Use of the VA (8%) and police (12%) were the least frequently reported services. On average, older LGBT adults used 1.7 services in this category.

HIV-related services and ASOs. The most frequently used services in this group were HIV services from the COH (23%), AIDS Foundation of Chicago (20%), Howard Brown Health Services (19%). Smaller proportions used the Test Positive Aware Network (14%) and the CORE center (10%) or Chicago House and Social Services (10%), whereas use of Better Existence with HIV (BEHIV) was reported by 9% of the sample. Five percent or fewer reported using the South Side Help Center of the Chicago Women's AIDS Project. Because nearly all the HIV-positive individuals in this sample were men, significantly greater proportions of men compared to women reported using the AIDS Foundation of Chicago, BEHIV, the Test Positive Aware Network, and the CORE Center (see Table 4). Use of services in this domain was significantly higher among men ($M = 1.5$) as compared with women ($M = 0.4$).

Health and long-term care services. The most frequently utilized service in this area was the dentist/dental clinic, with nearly one-half of older LGBT respondents reporting such use in the past year. Outpatient hospital care was reported by 38%, whereas 19% had received inpatient hospital care (see Table 4). Over one-fourth had used the hospital emergency room in the past year. One-third reported going to a private medical clinic and 1 out of 10 had utilized a Health Maintenance Organization. Behavioral health and substance use treatments were also utilized, with 27% having received mental health treatment and 11% utilizing drug or alcohol treatment and recovery programs. Case management, was reported by nearly one-third of participants (29%). Twice as many men had used case management (33%) as compared with women (16%). This is likely due to the proportion of HIV+ men in the sample as we also found that HIV+ older LGBT adults were significantly more likely to use case management (61%) as compared to their peers (12%). Few older LGBT adults had accessed homecare services (17%) or institutional long-term or continuing care (5%). Three percent used hospice during the previous year. On average, older LGBT adults used 2.6 health or long-term care services.

Other community-based organizations (CBOs). Senior centers were the most frequently used community-based service (25%). Clergy, meal and nutrition programs, and legal services were used by about one out of five older LGBT adults during the previous year (23%, 21% and 20%, respectively). Approximately 15% had attended a self-help group in the past year. In this group, only one significant gender difference emerged; older gay and bisexual men were significantly more likely to have turned to clergy (27%) as compared with lesbian and bisexual women (8%). Older LGBT adults used 1.0 of such CBO services, on average.

Use of services provided by the COH. Participants were asked about services provided by COH. The most frequently utilized service provided by COH was the Senior Congregate Meal Program (36%). The COH's Senior Social and Education programs were the next most frequently used (28%), followed by the computer technology center (26%). Approximately 1 out of 10 had had used the COH HIV support group (10%), mental health supportive services (11%) and legal services (11%). The only significant gender differences observed werer that older men were more likely to have used the HIV support group (14%) and legal assistance (13%) as compared with women (0% and 2%, respectively). The average number of COH services used was 1.1.

Need for Services in the Previous Year

Older LGBT adults were asked about their service needs in the past year from a list of commonly utilized health and social services (see Table 5). The average number of services needed in the past year was 2.5. In terms of specific service needs, socialization opportunities were among the most frequently mentioned with 51% of older LGBT adults indicating needing someplace to socialize (see Table 5). The need for a regular contact, either by a visit in person or by phone, was indicated by one-fourth of older LGBT adults. Regarding social service needs, counseling assistance, either personal or family, was the third highest in terms of need in the previous year (29%). Help navigating the entitlement system was an expressed need for 23% of older LGBT adults in the past year. Eighteen percent of older LGBT adults reported that they had needed help finding a job in the past year. With regard to household-related services, the most frequently reported service need in this domain was help with home repairs, which was reported by 23% of older LGBT adults. Nearly one out of five older LGBT adults reported that they had needed help with housekeeping or personal care in the home over the previous year (18%). Four percent of older LGBT adults reported that they needed meals brought to them at home during the previous year ($n = 8$; see Table 5). In the final domain of health-care related services, the most frequently reported need was assistance in getting to the doctor's office or a medical clinic (32%). Approximately one out of five (21%) older LGBT adults reported needing help following a stay in the hospital in the previous year. The need for homecare services (i.e., visiting nurse, home health aide, or home attendant) was reported by 12% of older LGBT adults.

There were few gender differences with regard to service needs in the previous year (see Table 5). Older gay and bisexual men were significantly more likely than women to mention they needed help navigating the entitlement system (27% and 12%, respectively), likely due to the preponderance of HIV cases in the former group. In fact, those with an HIV diagnosis were significantly more likely than their peers to indicate a need for this type of assistance (40% and 14%, respectively). Men were more than twice as likely to indicate that they needed help finding a job (21%) compared with women (8%). Finally, over one-third of lesbian and bisexual women indicated that they needed help with home repairs (35%), significantly higher as compared to men (19%).

Qualitative Analysis of Unmet Needs for Services

Using a grounded-theory approach (Glaser & Strauss, 1967), we identified 35 individual themes based on two open-ended questions concerning (a) unmet needs and (b) additional services desired at COH. Because of the extent of overlap in responses, we combined these data for the analyses reported in the following. Individual themes were grouped into four "families" (i.e., superordinate themes) that represented (a) needing help with basic support and instrumental tasks (b) education and recreation services, (c) health-related services, and (d) social services (see Table 6).

TABLE 6 List of Code Families and Codes From Qualitative Analysis of Unmet Service Needs

Needed Services			
Help With Support or Instrumental Tasks	Education or Recreation Programs	Health-Related	Social Services
Help with household tasks (1)	Computer or technology (3)	CAM (1)	Caregiving support (1)
Home repairs (3)	Culinary (2)	Dental care (5)	Case manager (1)
Nutrition program (6)	Cultural (1)	Health or medical care (2)	Employment or job placement (19)
	Education (2)	HIV/AIDS services at COH (2)	Entitlement or insurance help (5)
	LGBT discussion group (1)	Medication adherence and support (1)	Financial help/planning (10)
	Spanish language (1)	Mental health (3)	Friendly visiting (1)
	Spiritual or religious activities (3)	Non-HIV related LGBT services (1)	Gay parents group (1)
	Sports and recreation (6)	Substance abuse recovery (3)	Homeless services (3)
	Volunteer opportunities (1)	Vision care (1)	Housing/senior housing (21)
			Legal services (6)
			Lonely/isolated (5)
			Senior/senior programs at COH (1)
			Socialization opportunities (17)
			Support/education groups (2)

Note. Frequency of quotations (*n*). LGBT = lesbian, gay, bisexual, and transgender; CAM = complementary and alternative medicine; COH = Center on Halsted.

Help with basic support and instrumental tasks. Although relatively young (i.e., average age 60 years), many needed basic supports and help with instrumental tasks. Home repairs were a problem, as illustrated by a 66-year-old woman who shared that her son was too busy to help her with home maintenance. Others described more basic needs, such as the 59-year-old man who reported, "I have trouble getting around, getting food." Others said they were in need of nutrition programs or an increase in their food stamp benefits.

Education and recreation services. There was interest in a wide range of educational and recreational programs, including computer and technology classes, and culinary programs. A 60-year-old woman suggested that financial barriers exist in accessing culture and the arts wanting "more affordable cultural programs." Some wanted educational programs, or programs to assist with returning to school. A 63-year-old man was interested in a LGBT-identified discussion group, but was concerned about feeling shy and feared rejection. Spiritual and religious programs were wanted, specifically programs that did not discriminate based on sexual identity. General sports and recreation programs were mentioned, with interests ranging from sports, to yoga and exercise classes, and board and card games.

Health-related services. Some older LGBT adults were interested in complementary and alternative medicine, such as acupuncture. Others wanted adherence programs for HIV medication, but a 50-year-old woman wanted to see more non-HIV specific health services. Dental care was frequently reported, with many citing the lack of Medicare coverage for such services. Mental health and substance abuse recovery services were also mentioned frequently. A 56-year-old Black man described how the need for mental health services was related to cultural issues:

> For Afro-American [sic], it is in our culture not to seek help for depression or marital/family decisions. We need to learn that talking to a counselor or psychiatrist or taking meds for depression does not mean you are looney [sic] tunes (crazy).

Social services. Older LGBT respondents needed a wide range social services (see Table 6). Three areas stood out: employment assistance, housing, and socialization opportunities. Given the severe economic recession and high levels of unemployment during the time of data collection (i.e., 2010–2011), it was not surprising that help finding a job and employment counseling were needed. Some reported that they had been looking for work but were not successful. Many indicated that job-seeking efforts were hampered by ageism. A 60-year-old man related, "There are not jobs for people over 50 and no one is working to address that specific need!" Another 57-year-old woman said, " . . . for any leads I get, the employer is always looking for someone younger."

Given the high cost of living in urban areas like Chicago, it was not surprising that many were seeking affordable housing. A 73-year-old man told us, "Right now I need subsidized housing. My apartment had a fire and right now I'm kind of homeless and staying with friends." A number of individuals were interested in senior or supportive housing for older adults, many wanting a gay-friendly or a LGBT-focused facility. The third major area of unmet needs concerned opportunities for socialization, often motivated by feelings of loneliness and isolation. A 51-year-old transgender woman described how her substance abuse treatment created barriers to socialization that she wished to overcome:

> My social network outside of the [I]nternet has been limited to rehab, half-way house, sober living housing and respite shelter. I need a social life with regular people in the outside world.

Although the bar scene has been a social staple for the LGBT community, a common remark by the older respondents in this sample was a need for venues outside of this domain. One 54-year-old woman said, "Don't know where to go besides clubs to meet people. Want a girlfriend." Noting the ageism that persists in LGBT communities, a 67-year-old man told us, "I feel lonely and isolated a lot of the time (partly internalized ageism). I don't know where to go to meet other gay men my own age in a healthy setting, not bar, etc." Many lesbian and bisexual women related the difficulties they had on the social scene as they got older:

> Lesbians have limited social environments after age 50. Bar scene, limited at best, is for younger women. Fundraisers are too costly ($300 for date and me to go to Lesbian Community Care Project). Social events give 50+ women chance to meet other women, reconnect with friends, etc. (50-year-old woman).

Another important issue for older LGBT adults was needed assistance with either entitlement or insurance, or with regard to financial help/planning. A 56-year-old man told us, "I worry about surviving financially until I'm eligible for Social Security." Financial issues involved financial planning, as well as the need for financial assistance. A 50-year-old Black woman wanted "bankruptcy (or housing) help for those LGBTs affected by the economy." A number of respondents indicated a need for direct financial help and support. One man (age unknown) shared the difficulties he faced living on disability checks:

> Anybody on SSI or SSDI should be qualified for all services because that is not a living amount of money—it is only maintaining you. No money for trips or special places to go. Nothing left over. From month to month.

Summary of qualitative findings. The preceding qualitative analysis of the service needs of older LGBT adults has reinforced the quantitative information given by these respondents. But, more important, it has revealed additional areas of unmet need in this population. What was striking was the need for many of these respondents for basic human requirements such as food, shelter, or a viable occupation to provide economic security. Medical and dental care needs were mentioned by many, with lack of insurance coverage serving as a significant barrier. Isolation and socialization opportunities were also prominent. Socializing and finding romantic partners appeared to be a particular challenge for older lesbians, but the problem of ageism in the LGBT community was cited by both women and men. However, there was a significant amount of need expressed by these older adults for educational and recreational programs leading to self-improvement and enjoyment and highlighting positive aspects of LGBT aging.

DISCUSSION

This study of the social care networks of older LGBT adults in Chicago extends the limited research in this domain with regard to social support networks and exchanges of assistance, and contributes new findings in the areas of service utilization and the service needs of this population. Although this sample reported relatively high socioeconomic status in terms of education and income adequacy, it is important to recognize that many were struggling economically with nearly one out of six not having enough for expenses. Nearly one-half were just managing on their incomes, dispelling the myth of the "wealthy" gay demographic, echoing other research on income disparities in this population (Black, Makar, Sanders, & Taylor, 2003; Martell, 2010; Prokos & Keene, 2010). HIV has clearly had an impact on this community and contributed to the high rates of disability (30%) and the high prevalence of physical and mental health conditions. However, HIV is not the only health issue for this group. On average, the number of health conditions among those without HIV was 2.4 as compared to 2.6 for the entire sample (i.e., including those with HIV). Among those who are HIV-positive, an average of 3.1 comorbid conditions is reported, nearly identical to the findings on HIV-positive adults over 50 in New York (Havlik et al., 2011). Approximately one out of six reported at least one PADL difficulty, whereas over one-third had at least one IADL challenge. One-third had rates of depressive symptoms considered to be clinically significant. Smoking and substance use were also prevalent. These findings on the physical and mental health status of this population reflect data from other reports (Fredriksen-Goldsen et al., 2011; IOM, 2011).

Considering their relatively young average age of 60 years, the findings on health and disability rates in this sample suggest that many will need to engage their social care networks now and in the future. Only one-third have spouses or partners, and nearly two-thirds live alone. Men were significantly more likely to report living alone than women and are likely at greatest risk for isolation, as has been documented in other studies (Fredriksen-Goldsen et al., 2011; Grossman et al., 2000; Shippy et al., 2004). Although the biological family is present, many family members are not connected with these LGBT older adults and cannot be classified as functional members of the social care system. Lesbian and bisexual women are significantly more likely to have children and grandchildren, and are also more likely to keep in contact with siblings compared with men. Consequently, women appeared to benefit from their greater likelihood of having offspring in terms of significantly larger social networks and receiving more types of help from family members compared to men. However, this greater involvement with family often translated into increased levels of negative social support.

Congruent with other research on LGBT populations, friends are the backbone of the social support networks, and were the most prevalent functional network element (77%). Research has found that older LGBT adults who report having friends available for needed assistance evidence better mental health compared to their counterparts without such support (Masini & Barrett, 2008; Shippy et al., 2004; Smith, McCaslin, Chang, Martinez, & McGrew, 2010). Indeed, we found that in this sample, having a functional friend was correlated with positive affect ($r = .16$, $p < .02$) and depression ($r = −.16$, $p < .02$). Older gay and bisexual men had significantly more friends with HIV when compared to women ($M = 1.1$ and $M = 0.2$, respectively). This may have consequences for these older men as they attempt to secure caregiving and other supports as they grow older. Because HIV-positive older adults have high rates of morbidity and resultant functional incapacity, these friends may not be in a position to provide support in times of need.

Reflecting Cantor's Hierarchical Compensatory Theory of social supports (see Cantor & Mayer, 1978) and their social network characteristics, older LGBT adults reported frequently turning to formal community-based services, using approximately six, on average, in the previous year. Gay and bisexual men, who were more likely to be HIV-positive and use HIV services, reported higher service use overall compared with women. This finding is explained by two factors; need and the use of case management. As noted earlier, those with HIV in this sample and a greater number of comorbid conditions, on average, compared to their peers, and thus likely have higher service needs. Other research has documented that higher levels of need tend to drive service utilization in older populations (Brennan-Ing, Seidel, London, Cahill, & Karpiak, 2014/this issue; Cantor & Brennan, 1993, 2000). In addition, the HIV-positive participants in this sample are also more likely to have used case management services compared to those without an

HIV diagnosis (61% and 12%, respectively; Brennan-Ing, Karpiak, & Seidel, 2011). Higher utilization of case management is also linked greater service utilization (Brennan-Ing et al., 2014/this issue; Cunningham, Wong, & Hays, 2008; London, LeBlanc, & Aneshensel, 1998). In terms of other services, older gay and bisexual men were almost 3 times as likely as women to have sought assistance from religious clergy in the past year. This may also be explained by the higher prevalence of HIV among men in this sample. HIV infection, although currently a treatable illness, remains life-altering and life-threatening and may lead one to seek religious and spiritual guidance in coping and adjusting to this diagnosis (Brennan, 2008; Vance, Brennan, Enah, Smith, & Kaur, 2011).

Older LGBT adults reported needing, on average, 2.5 services in the previous year. More men than women reported needing help with entitlements or finding a job, which is in line with the higher rates of disability and lower rates of employment in this sample among men as compared with women. Women were more likely to say they needed help with home repairs (35%), which was also an issue for one out of five men. This is congruent with the greater likelihood of lesbian and bisexual women in this sample to be co-op or condominium owners compared to gay and bisexual men (63% and 37%, respectively).

A majority of the sample reported the need for socialization opportunities. As noted earlier, nearly two-thirds of this sample lived alone, which fosters social isolation and feelings of loneliness. In addition, the qualitative findings revealed that, although gay and lesbian bars are often the public squares of the LGBT community, many of these older adults were looking for other venues to meet friends and romantic interests. Part of this was due to the perceived ageism in the bar scene, and part was not knowing what other options were available.

Many of these LGBT adults see aging as chance to grow, explore and make the most of life. Although our quantitative inquiry had focused on health and social service needs, a number of respondents used the open-ended items to express the need for educational, cultural, and recreational programs. Cost was clearly an issue for a number of individuals and financial help in accessing these resources was expressed. There was also unmet need expressed for spiritual and religious programs that would respect their sexual and gender identities.

Limitations

This study employed a convenience sample of older LGBT adults and the extent to which the findings are generalizable to the larger population are unknown. Due to small numbers, we were unable to perform statistical comparisons with transgender or intersex respondents, although they were included in the overall descriptive data and qualitative analysis. Future research should specifically target these groups and recruit samples of a sufficient size to yield valid data. Finally, the bivariate comparisons made between men and women did not control for other factors on which these two groups differ. However, because our purpose was to provide information useful for policy and program planning, we felt the comparison by gender was both useful and appropriate.

Program Implications

Many aging LGBT adults will likely need to access community-based services given their high levels of need and often inadequate or unavailable informal social supports. How will the current network of aging service providers rise to meet this challenge? At present, LGBT older adults needing formal assistance may access services tailored to the LGBT community or seek mainstream aging services; both have challenges. LGBT-specific social services are unavailable in many communities. For example, Knochel et al. (2011) found that only 2% of aging service providers offered gay- and lesbian-specific services. Another study found that only a little more than 10% of substance abuse treatment centers had services tailored for the LGBT population (A. K. Hughes et al., 2011). Nationally, few older LGBT adults have access to services addressing their specific needs. In large metropolitan areas such as Chicago, there tends to be greater availability of programs such as the senior programs at the COH. Although it was only this year that SAGE was able to establish the first LGBT-dedicated senior center in New York City, despite the historically large sexual minority population in the area (SAGE, 2013b). However, even in large urban areas, services may not be available as one respondent in this study noted the dearth of LGBT providers on Chicago's South Side. Clearly we need to expand local programs and other opportunities that specifically target LGBT older adults in the communities where they reside.

Findings from this study underscore that some LGBT older adults do rely on LGBT-focused organizations to meet their needs, yet they tend to mainly rely on mainstream providers, such as government offices and agencies (1.7 services, on average), community-based social support, and health care providers (2.6 services, on average). However, challenges exist for older LGBT adults when trying to access mainstream services. Some fear doing so due to real and perceived discrimination (Knochel et al., 2011). Accessing mainstream providers also raises the issue of sexual identity disclosure to non-LGBT providers, which is exacerbated by fear of discrimination. This was supported by our qualitative data specifically around accessing religious and spiritual programs. For mainstream service providers, identifying and working with the older LGBT population, which can be "invisible" is a challenge. Disclosure to health care providers is critical to receiving appropriate care and it has been suggested that routine questions about sexual identity could assist in this process. However, studies have demonstrated that non-disclosure to health providers is not uncommon (Clover, 2006; Steele, Tinmouth, & Lu, 2006; Wilging, Salvador, & Kano, 2006). In addition, disclosure appears to be more difficult for lesbians, as well as gay and bisexual men of color (Bernstein et al., 2008; Klitzman & Greenberg, 2002).

Without a concerted effort to address the unique issues of LGBT aging and to intentionally create a safe and welcoming space for LGBT older adults, it remains likely that LGBT older adults may be reluctant to access mainstream services. Thus, it is imperative that mainstream providers improve their LGBT cultural competency through training and capacity building efforts. Some interventions have focused on the creation of more culturally competent LGBT services by sensitizing health and aging providers through the use of education directed at staff and engaging the LGBT community; however, the effectiveness of these programs was mixed (Anetzberger, Ishler, Mustade, & Blair, 2004; Clark, Landers, Linde, & Sperber, 2001). On the positive side, many aging providers are open to receiving such training and better serving older LGBT adults (Knochel et al., 2011). Given the mixed-results to date, it is important that such programs be evaluated in terms of efficacy and best practices. LGBT cultural competency should be mandated for providers receiving local, state, or federal funding.

Finally, specific steps must be taken at the program level to address the socialization needs and pervasive isolation that too often characterize the aging LGBT adult. Isolation contributes to feelings of loneliness and depression, which, in turn, are related to poorer heath outcomes (Havlik et al., 2011). Moreover, isolation reduces the already frail support systems of these LGBT older adults because it mitigates against their ability to cultivate additional support resources as they grow older. There are many steps programs can take to reduce isolation. For example at COH, isolation is reduced by connecting individuals with their peers through a variety of social, recreational and educational programs specifically designed for LGBT older adults.

Policy Implications

Population-based LGBT research. Findings from this study underscore the challenges that older LGBT adults confront as they age with regard to financial difficulties and physical illness. More must be done to better document the health and economic disparities faced by LGBT adults as they age. At present, there is no representative national survey or database available to inform us on this topic (IOM, 2011). The inclusion of sexual orientation and gender identity questions on national surveys is crucial if we are to obtain sound population-based data on LGBT older adults, and the U.S. HHS (2011) is taking important steps in this direction.

Housing. The need for senior housing that addressed the unique needs of the LGBT community was frequently expressed in our qualitative data. This may reflect fear of discrimination and poor treatment in mainstream environs. Affordable housing was also a concern for the older LGBT adults in this study. Federal support for senior housing, such as Section 8, should in part focus on developing and identifying affordable LGBT senior housing. In addition, Title VIII of the *Civil Rights Act of 1968* (Fair Housing Act; U.S. Department of Housing and Urban Development, 2013) should be expanded to prohibit housing discrimination against LGBT adults.

Older Americans Act reauthorization. Declaring older LGBT adults a population of "greatest social need" would help to direct federal monies supporting state and local area agencies on aging to meet the health, housing, economic, and social service needs of this population. This would also assist in freeing funding for urgently needed cultural competency programs for aging providers.

CONCLUSION

Whereas aging is a time of personal growth for some, other older LGBT adults face considerable challenges in meeting basic human needs. Some had trouble being able to afford and secure food. Chronic health issues are common in this population and suggest that caregiving and other forms of assistance will be necessary to enable many of these individuals to continue to live independently. Although considerable support is received from friends, the majority live alone, and many lack the family supports that most older adults rely on in times of need. Unemployment in this group was higher than the national average (12%) and many had difficulties finding a job, often due to apparent ageism. Others had a need for affordable housing suitable to older adults, or were in fact homeless. Some of these older adults who identify these basic needs are utilizing government and community-based services and are likely receiving entitlements, but they perceive that the safety net is fraying and their quality of life has begun to decline. For those who are isolated due to illness, stigma or an absence of friends and family members, the risk is that these older LGBT adults will fall through the cracks if we are unable to better address their social care needs.

FUNDING

Funding for this study was obtained from a grant from Human Resources Services Administration to the Center on Halsted, Chicago, IL, who commissioned the work with AIDS Community Research Initiative of America.

REFERENCES

American Lung Association. (2010). *Smoking out a deadly threat: Tobacco use in the LGBT community.* Retrieved November 4, 2013 from http://www.lung.org/assets/documents/publications/lung-disease-data/lgbt-report.pdf

Andersen, E. M., Malmgren, J. A., Carter, W. B., & Patrick, D. L. (1994). Screening for depression in well older adults: Evaluation of a short form of the CES–D (Center for Epidemiologic Studies Depression Scale). *American Journal of Preventative Medicine, 10,* 77–84.

Anetzberger, G. J., Ishler, K. J., Mustade, J., & Blair, M. (2004). Gray and gay: A community dialogue on issues and concerns of older gays and lesbians. *Journal of Gay and Lesbian Social Services, 17,* 23–24.

Bernstein, K. T., Liu, K. L., Begier, E. M., Koblin, B., Karpati, A., & Murrill, C. (2008). Same-sex attraction disclosure to health care providers among New York City men who have sex with men. *Archive of Internal Medicine, 168,* 1458–1464.

Black, D. A., Makar, H. R., Sanders, S. G., & Taylor, L. J. (2003). The earnings effects of sexual orientation. *Industrial & Labor Relations Review, 56*(3). Retrieved from http://digitalcommons.ilr.cornell.edu/ilrreview/vol56/iss3/5

Brennan, M. (2008). Older men living with HIV: The importance of spirituality. *Generations, 32*(1), 54–61.

Brennan, M., Karpiak, S. E., Shippy, R. A., & Cantor, M. H. (Eds.). (2009). *Older adults with HIV: An in-depth examination of an emerging population.* New York, NY: Nova Science.

Brennan-Ing, M., Karpiak, S. E., & Seidel, L. (2011). *Health and psychosocial needs of LGBT older adults. Final report to the Center on Halsted, Chicago, IL.* New York, NY: AIDS Community Research of America, Center on HIV and Aging.

Brotman, S., Ryan, B., & Cormier, R. (2003). The health and service needs of gay and lesbian elders and their families in Canada. *Gerontologist, 43,* 192–202.

Cantor, M. H., & Brennan, M. (1993). *Family and community support systems of older New Yorkers. Growing older in New York City in the 1990s: A study of changing lifestyles, quality of life, and quality of care, Vol. V.* New York, NY: New York Center for Policy on Aging, New York Community Trust.

Cantor, M. H., & Brennan, M. (2000). *Social care of the elderly: The effects of ethnicity, class and culture.* New York, NY: Springer.

Cantor, M. H., Brennan, M., & Shippy, R. A. (2004). *Caregiving among older lesbian, gay, bisexual, and transgender New Yorkers. Final report.* Washington, DC: National Gay and Lesbian Task Force Policy Institute.

Cantor, M. H., & Mayer, M. (1978). Factors in differential utilization of services by urban elderly. *Journal of Gerontological Social Work, 1*(1), 47–61.

Centers for Disease Control and Prevention. (2010). Diagnoses of HIV infection and AIDS in the United States and dependent areas, 2010. *HIV Surveillance Report, 22.* Retrieved from http://www.cdc.gov/hiv/surveillance/resources/reports/2010report/index.htm

Clark, M. E., Landers, S., Linde, R., & Sperber, J. (2001). The GLBT health access project: A state-funded effort to improve access to care. *American Journal of Public Health, 91,* 895–896.

Clover, D. (2006). Overcoming barriers for older gay men in the use of health services: A qualitative study of growing older, sexuality and health. *Health Education Journal, 65*(1), 41–52.

Cunningham, W. E., Wong, M., & Hays, R. D. (2008). Case management and health-related quality of life outcomes in a national sample of persons with HIV/AIDS. *Journal of the National Medical Association, 100*, 840–847.

de Vries, B., & Hoctel, P. (2007). The family friends of older gay men and lesbians. In N. Teunis & G. Herdt (Eds.), *Sexual inequalities and social justice* (pp. 213–232). Berkeley, CA: University of California Press.

Dorfman, R., Walters, K., Burke, P., Hardin, L., & Karanik, T. (1995). Old, sad and alone: The myth of the aging homosexual. *Journal of Gerontological Social Work, 24*(1/2), 29–44.

Effros, R., Fletcher, C., Gebo, K., Halter, J. B., Hazzard, W., Horne, F., . . .High K. P. (2008). Workshop on HIV infection and aging: What is known and future research directions. *Clinical Infectious Diseases, 47*, 542–553.

Fillenbaum, G. G. (1988). *Multidimensional functional assessment of older adults: The Duke Older Americans Resources and Services procedures.* Hillsdale, NJ: Erlbaum.

Fredriksen-Goldsen, K. I., Kim, H. J., Emlet, C. A., Muraco, A., & Erosheva, E. (2011). *The aging and health report: Disparities and resilience among lesbian, gay, bisexual, and transgender older adults.* Seattle, WA: Institutional for Multigenerational Health.

Glaser, B., & Strauss, A. (1967). *The discovery of grounded theory.* Chicago, IL: Aldine.

Grossman, A. H., D'Augelli, A. R., & Hershberger, S. L. (2000). Social support networks of lesbian, gay and bisexual adults 60 years of age and older. *Journal of Gerontology: Psychological Sciences, 55B*(3), P171–P179.

Havlik, R. J., Brennan, M., & Karpiak, S. E. (2011). Comorbidities and depression in older adults with HIV. *Sexual Health, 8*, 551–559. doi:10.1071/SH11017

Hughes, A. K., Harold, R. D., & Boyer, J. M. (2011). Awareness of LGBT aging issues among aging services network providers. *Journal of Gerontological Social Work, 54*, 659–677.

Hughes, M. (2007). Older lesbians and gays accessing health and aged-care services. *Australian Social Work, 60*, 197–209.

Institute of Medicine. (2011). *The health of lesbian, gay, bisexual, and transgender people: Building a foundation for better understanding.* Washington, DC: National Academies Press.

Israel, T., Walther, W., Gortcheva, R., & Perry, J. S. (2011). Policies and practices for LGBT clients: Perspectives of mental health services administrators. *Journal of Gay and Lesbian Mental Health Providers, 15*, 152–168.

Klitzman, R., & Greenberg, J. (2002). Patterns of communication between gay and lesbian patients and their health care providers. *Journal of Homosexuality, 42*(4), 65–75.

Knochel, K. A., Quam, J. K., & Croghan, C. F. (2011). Are old lesbian and gay people well served? Understanding the perceptions, preparation, and experiences of aging services providers. *Journal of Applied Gerontology, 30*, 370–389.

Lindau, S. T., Schumm, L. P., Laumann, E. O. , Levinson, W., O'Muircheartaigh, C. A., & Waite, L. J. (2007). A study of sexuality and health among older adults in the United States. *New England Journal of Medicine, 357,* 762–774.

London, A. S., LeBlanc, A. J., & Aneshensel, C. S. (1998). The integration of informal care, case management, and community-based services for people with HIV. *AIDS Care, 21,* 874–880.

Martell, M. E. (2010). *Why do homosexual men earn less than heterosexual men, despite an invisible minority trait?* Retrieved from http://www.american.edu/cas/economics/pdf/upload/Paper-Martell.pdf

Masini, B. E., & Barrett, H. A. (2008). Social support as a predictor of psychological and physical well-being and lifestyle in lesbian, gay, and bisexual adults aged 50 and over. *Journal of Gay and Lesbian Social Services, 20,* 91–110.

Muhr, T. (1997). ATLAS.ti for Windows: Visual qualitative data analysis, management, & model building [Computer software]. Berlin, Germany: Scientific Software Development.

Prokos, A. H., & Keene, J. R. (2010). Poverty among cohabitating gay and lesbian, and married and cohabitating heterosexual families. *Journal of Family Issues, 31,* 934–959.

Radloff, L. S. (1977). The CES–D scale: A self-report depression scale for research in the general population. *Applied Psychological Measurement, 1,* 385–401.

Services and Advocacy for GLBT Elders (SAGE). (2013a). *National resource center on LGBT aging.* Retrieved from http://www.sageusa.org/programs/nrc.cfm

Services and Advocacy for GLBT Elders (SAGE). (2013b). *The SAGE center.* Retrieved November 4, 2013 from http://www.sageusa.org/nyc/thesagecenter.cfm

Sheehan, N. W., Wilson, R., & Marella, L. M. (1988). The role of church in providing services for the aging. *Journal of Applied Gerontology, 7,* 231–241.

Shippy, R. A., Cantor, M. H., & Brennan, M. (2004). Social networks of aging gay men. *Journal of Men's Studies, 13*(1), 107–120.

Smith, L. A., McCaslin, R., Chang, J., Martinez, P., & McGrew, P. (2010). Assessing the needs of older gay, lesbian, bisexual and transgender people: A service-learning and agency partnership approach. *Journal of Gerontological Social Work, 53,* 387–401.

Steele, L., Tinmouth, J. M., & Luc, A. (2006). Regular care use by lesbians: A path analysis of predictive factors. *Family Practice, 23,* 631–636.

Stein, G. L., & Bonuck, K. A. (2001). Attitudes on end-of-life care and advance care planning in the lesbian and gay community. *Journal of Palliative Medicine, 4,* 173–190.

Substance Abuse and Mental Health Services Administration. (2012). *Top health issues for LGBT populations information & resource kit* (Department of Health and Human Services Pub. No. SMA 12-4684). Rockville, MD: Author.

Tan, P. P. (2005). The importance of spirituality among gay and lesbian individuals. *Journal of Homosexuality, 49*(2), 135–144.

Tirrito, T., & Choi, G. (2005). Faith organizations and ethnically diverse elders: A community-action model. *Journal of Religious Gerontology, 16,* 123–142.

Tjepkema, M. (2008). Health care use among gay, lesbian and bisexual Canadians. *Health Reports, 19*(1), 53–64.

U.S. Department of Health and Human Services. (2010). *Healthy People 2020* (Office of Disease Prevention and Human Promotion Pub. No. B0132). Washington, DC: Author.

U.S. Department of Health and Human Services. (2011). *Affordable Care Act to improve data collection, reduce health disparities.* Washington, DC: Author. Retrieved from http://www.hhs.gov/news/press/2011pres/06/20110629a.html

U.S. Department of Housing and Urban Development (HUD). (2013). *The Fair Housing Act.* Retrieved November 4, 2013 from http://portal.hud.gov/hudportal/HUD?src=/program_offices/fair_housing_equal_opp/progdesc/title8

Vance, D. E., Brennan, M., Enah, C., Smith, G. L., & Kaur, J. (2011). Religion, spirituality, and older adults with HIV: Critical personal and social resources for an aging epidemic. *Clinical Interventions in Aging, 6,* 101–109.

Wallace, S. P., Cochran, S. D., Durazo, E. M., & Ford, C. L. (2011). *The health of aging lesbian, gay and bisexual adults in California.* Los Angeles, CA: UCLA Center for Health Policy Research.

Wilging, C. E., Salvador, M., & Kano, M. (2006). Pragmatic help seeking: How sexual and gender minority groups access mental health care in a rural state. *Psychiatric Services, 57,* 871–874.

Investigating the Needs and Concerns of Lesbian, Gay, Bisexual, and Transgender Older Adults: The Use of Qualitative and Quantitative Methodology

NANCY A. OREL, PhD, LPC

Gerontology Program, Bowling Green State University, Bowling Green, Ohio, USA

Extensive research on the specific needs and concerns of lesbian, gay, bisexual, and transgender (LGBT) older adults is lacking. This article describes the results of both quantitative studies (i.e., LGBT Elders Needs Assessment Scale) and qualitative studies (i.e., focus groups and in-depth interviews with lesbian, gay, or bisexual [LGB] older adults and LGB grandparents) that specifically sought to investigate the unique needs and concerns of LGBT elders. The results identified 7 areas (medical/health care, legal, institutional/housing, spiritual, family, mental health, and social) of concern and the recognition that the needs and concerns of LGBT older adults be addressed across multiple domains, rather than in isolation.

It is well documented that the population over the age of 65 within the United States and worldwide is dramatically increasing. While the overall U.S. population has tripled in the past century, the number of people aged 65 and older has increased 11-fold (Administration on Aging, 2010; U.S. Census Bureau, 2000). Currently, nearly 35 million Americans are aged 65 and older, representing 13% of the population, or one in eight Americans. During the next 25 years, as baby boomers reach later life, the number of American elders will almost double to 69.4 million. The accelerated pace of the aging population is most evident with the fact that beginning on January 1, 2011, approximately 10,000 "baby boomers" (e.g., those born between the years 1946 and 1964) will turn age 65 each day. It is estimated that in 2030, one in five Americans will be 65 years of age or older. Because life expectancy has increased, the number of individuals reaching the age of 85 or older will also dramatically increase. It is projected that by 2050, the United States may have as many people over the age of 85 as the current populations of New York City, Los Angeles, and Chicago combined (Administration on Aging, 2010).

Paralleling the overall older adult population, it can be assumed that the number and proportion of lesbian, gay, bisexual, and transgender (LGBT) older adults will significantly increase over the next few decades. However, obtaining accurate estimations of the current and projected LGBT older adult population has been problematic for a variety of reasons, but mostly due to the fact that sexual orientation has been absent in almost all major gerontological research studies (Barranti & Cohen, 2000), especially federal surveys (Institute of Medicine, 2011). In addition, the pervasive homophobic attitudes of society have discouraged the LGBT older adult population from "coming out" and being counted (Hunter, 2007). Therefore, only rough estimations of the LGBT older adult population are presently available. These estimations are based on historical estimates of the overall LGBT population, which have ranged from as low as 1% to as high as 10% of the general population (D'Augelli & Patterson, 1996; Kinsey, Pomeroy, & Martin, 1948; Kochman, 1997). Recently, publications from both the Institute of Medicine (2011) and the Williams Institute (Gates, 2011) indicate that determining the size of the LGBT population remains challenging, but using available data, they estimate that 3.5% of adults in the United States identify as lesbian, gay, or bisexual (LGB), and an estimated 0.3% are transgender. The National Gay and Lesbian Task Force (NGLTF) Policy Institute (1999) recommended the use of a conservative range of 3% to 8% to estimate the actual LGBT older adult population. Applying these percentages, the NGLTF Policy Institute estimates that one to three million Americans aged 65 and older are LGBT.

The "graying of America" demands societal attention to the challenges and opportunities of the general older adult population; this statement takes on a heightened importance with reference to the aging LGBT population whose specific needs and experiences remain largely unknown. Concomitant with this absence of information, many researchers have concluded that the needs of LGBT older adults have been ignored by most institutions in our society (Dorfman et al., 1995; Quam & Whitford, 1992). In 2000, the NGLTF published *Outing Age*, the first comprehensive report to address public policy issues facing LGBT elders (Cahill, South, & Spade, 2000), with an updated version published in 2010 (Grant, Koskovick, Frazer, & Bjerk, 2010). In 2010, Services and Advocacy for GLBT Elders (SAGE) and the Movement Advancement Project in partnership with the American Society on Aging released *Improving the Lives of Lesbian, Gay, Bisexual, and Transgender Older Adults*. Most recently, the Institute of Medicine released in 2011

The Health of Lesbian, Gay, Bisexual, and Transgender People: Building a Foundation for Better Understanding. Collectively, these reports clearly indicate that research studies on LGBT older adults are desperately needed. The reports also stressed the importance of investigating the needs and concerns of middle-aged LGBT persons because there are distinguishable characteristics that differentiate midlife cohorts of LGBT individuals from current older cohorts.

For example, LGBT adults who are currently at the leading edge of the boomer cohort are the first generation to reach middle adulthood after the occurrence of the Stonewall riots in 1969 and the resulting gay liberation movement of the 1970s (Herdt & de Vries, 2004; Hunter, 2005: Richardson & Seidman, 2002). Current older cohorts of LGBT persons came of age during a significantly different sociohistorical context in which heterosexism went unchallenged and negative views toward homosexuality were made explicit throughout culture and social institutions (Hunter, 2005; Kimmel, Rose, Orel, & Greene, 2006). Prior to the Stonewall Rebellion of 1969, LGBT persons were forced to live secreted lives in which their sexual orientation was "closeted" so that a public heterosexual identity could be managed (Seidman, 2002).

This article, grouped into several studies adopting different methodologies, describes ongoing, linked research endeavors that have focused on the LGBT older adult population addressing the recommendations first made by the NGLTF in 2000. Specifically, our initial focus group discussions and individual interviews on needs and service usage led to the development of a needs assessment instrument, which, in turn, led to subsequent interviews on more focused topics. All of these research activities are presented collectively to represent the cumulative nature of this research and to illustrate the importance of conducting both quantitative and qualitative studies, and their mutual influence, to best address the research questions under consideration.

CONDUCTING FOCUS GROUPS WITH LGBT ELDERS

Historically, focus groups have been suggested as a useful starting point for the design of survey questionnaires (Stewart & Shamdasani, 1990). Maykut and Morehouse (1994) defined a focus group as "a group conversation with a purpose" (p. 104). Focus groups rely on group discussion and interaction that is based on the researcher's focus of inquiry (Morgan, 1997). The aim of this focus group research was to identify the common themes regarding the needs, concerns, and issues affecting a select group of older LGBT persons. It was believed that the identification of common themes would provide insights into focus group participants' attitudes, perceptions, and opinions about aging within the LGBT community and their utilization of aging services.

Three focus groups of 7 to 10 self-identified older LGB persons in three different geographical areas (Northwest, Ohio; Northeast, Ohio; and Southeast, Michigan) were organized and conducted. These three areas included three major metropolitan cities (e.g., Toledo, Cleveland, and Detroit), as well as suburban and rural communities that are diverse in terms of race and ethnicity. Following Institutional Human Subjects Review Board protocol, all focus group participants were informed, in writing, of the general nature of the research project, the foreseeable risks, and the voluntary nature of their participation.

A total of 26 LGB older adults participated in the focus group discussions. There were 13 lesbians, 10 gay men, and 3 women who identified their sexual orientation as bisexual. Unfortunately, the focus groups did not include older adults who self-identified as being transgender, despite vigorous recruitment efforts to be inclusive. Participants ranged in age from 65 to 84, with a mean age of 72.3. Collectively, the three focus groups consisted of LGB older adults of various ethnic and racial groups (African Americans, $n = 6$; European Americans, $n = 17$; Asian Americans, $n = 1$; Latino/Latinas, $n = 2$; socioeconomic statuses [low income, $n = 5$; middle income, $n = 15$; upper income, $n = 6$]) and educational levels (less than an 8th-grade education, $n = 2$; high school graduates, $n = 17$; college graduates, $n = 5$; advanced degrees, $n = 2$). The focus groups were conducted over a period of 6 months, and the length of each focus group was from $1\frac{1}{2}$ to 2 hr. All focus group discussions were audiotaped, and to protect the anonymity of the information that would be obtained, participants were asked to use pseudonyms instead of their own names. The physical locations of the focus group discussions were at pre-identified gay-friendly sites.

Audio-taped focus group discussions were transcribed verbatim. The qualitative analytic strategy that was used for the focus group transcripts was the constant comparative method suggested by Glaser and Strauss (1967), and further outlined by Maykut and Morehouse (1994). Transcripts underwent a process called "unitizing the data" (Maykut & Morehouse, 1994, p. 118) to identify units of meaning within the data. This process involved identifying small units of meaning, such that each unit of data that was identified was explicable by itself and later served as the basis for defining larger categories of meaning (Lincoln & Cuba, 1985).

The next step in the analysis process involved inductive category coding in which recurring ideas, themes, and concepts from the unitized data was combined into larger conceptual categories (Maykut & Morehouse, 1994; Merriam, 1998). Categories were continuously refined and reviewed for ambiguity or overlap. Taking these larger categories, salient patterns and relationships that emerged across categories were explored. The categorized and refined data were integrated into a descriptive narrative of the participating LGB older adults' experiences and perspectives (Maykut & Morehouse, 1994).

This descriptive content analysis of the expressed experiences, perspectives, attitudes, and opinions from participants in the three focus groups revealed seven major areas of importance for these LGB older adults. These seven areas (listed in order of implied importance by the participants) were medical/health care, legal, institutional/housing, spiritual, family, mental health, and social (Orel, 2004a). These seven life areas have also been previously identified in the literature as being areas of importance for *heterosexual* older men and women (Ferrini & Ferrini, 2000).

All focus group participants indicated that their medical/health care needs were their primary source of concern, with an emphasis on concerns related to rising health care costs, financial constraints in seeking medical care, and failing health. It was most evident from the focus group discussions that the health care needs of the LGB older adult participants mirrored what has been reported in previous studies (Dean et al., 2000; Gay and Lesbian Medical Association, 2001). There continues to be health disparities among LGBT persons, and LGBT elders specifically. Although a major goal that was highlighted in the Department of Health and Human Services' *Healthy People 2010* was the elimination of health disparities of LGBT individuals, research has suggested that LGBT persons are disproportionately at risk for violent hate crimes, sexually transmitted infections including HIV/AIDS, a variety of mental health conditions (Cochran, 2001; Cochran & Mays, 2000, 2009; Fergusson, Horwood, & Beautrais, 1999; Herek, 2009; Institute of Medicine, 2011; Koh & Ross, 2006), body weight problems (Carlat, Camargo, & Herzog, 1997; Carpenter, 2003; Deputy & Boehmer, 2010), substance use and abuse (Cochran & Mays, 2006; Skinner & Otis, 1996; Stall & Wiley, 1988), smoking (DuRant, Krowchuk, & Sinal, 1998; Stall et al., 1999; Tang et al., 2004), and certain cancers (Cochran et al., 2001; Daling et al., 1987; Dibble, Vanoni, & Miaskowski, 1997; Koblin et al., 1996; Zaritsky & Dibble, 2010). These same health risks were reported by members of the focus groups. That is, the discussions revealed patterns similar to previous research that indicates that lesbians are significantly less likely than non-lesbian women to receive routine preventive health care (e.g., pap smears and breast cancer screening; Denenberg, 1995; Institute of Medicine, 1999; Koh, 2000; Robertson & Schachter, 1981) and gay adults are significantly more likely than non-gay adults to report unmet medical needs and difficulty obtaining care (Diamanti, Schuster, & Lever, 2000; Diamanti, Wold, Spritzer, & Gelberg, 2000; Ponce et al., 2010). However, the exact causes of these health disparities are still understudied and, therefore, not well understood (Mayer et al., 2008). Meyer and Northridge (2007) suggested that the social stigma and systematic discrimination based on sexual orientation and gender identity create a stressful social environment that has a significant negative impact on the overall health of LGBT individuals. Focus group participants provided examples of the discrimination and bias that they experienced within health care settings. Participants shared their frustrations with health care personnel who would assume heterosexuality, especially when sexual histories were being obtained. More important, one-half of the participants indicated that their physicians did not discuss sexual activity or obtain sexual histories.

Legal issues were another identified source of primary concern and frustration for all twenty-six LGB elder focus group participants. Focus group participants voiced their frustrations about the lack of legal protection for same sex couples that "married" opposite sex couples are granted. Although focus groups participants discussed the availability of *living wills* and *durable power of attorney for health care,* they also provided specific examples of how these two documents are not sufficient for protecting their health concerns, especially in the provision of home health care and long-term institutional care. Focus group participants also expressed their hope that "things will get better" for future LGBT generations, especially if same sex relationships would be legally recognized.

This expression of hope for "things will get better" was also evident when LGB focus group participants discussed their experiences and willingness to disclose their sexual orientation to friends, family, or colleagues. The majority of focus group participants discussed how they experienced social stigma and systematic discrimination based both on their age and their sexual orientation. Focus group members discussed how issues related to housing, spirituality, mental health, family, and social networks intersected with both their age and sexual orientation. More specifically, focus group members identified that both ageism and heterosexism presented challenges when attempting to secure adequate housing and receive emotional/spiritual support. Likewise, many indicated that their ability to maintain supportive relationships with family and friends were becoming more challenging as they aged.

Many focus group members indicated that the strength of their past social networks and friendships was due to their ongoing involvement within the gay/lesbian community. The majority of participants indicated that their social networks were composed primarily of other LGBT individuals, but as they aged they recognized the limits of this exclusivity. As one participant said, "I don't want to be old and alone. When I lost all my gay friends to AIDS, I realized that my social sphere was pretty small. I can't just have gay friends" (Orel, 2004a, p. 68). Focus group members also questioned whether their current network of friends would be willing to assist them if they experienced some of their preconceived threats of old age (e.g., loneliness, isolation, failing health, and economic distress), and they questioned who would provide needed caregiving assistance because they do not have children. As one participant said, "Children are supposed to take care of their elders. What happens when you don't have children?" This comment led to an important topic of discussion for all focus group members: familial relationships and intergenerational relationships among LGBT older adults.

All focus group members discussed their familial relationships and ten members discussed their relationships with grown children from prior heterosexual relationships. Participants discussed how they "picked their battles" as far as disclosing their sexual orientation to siblings, grown children, and for some participants: their grandchildren. Focus group members' decision to disclose or remain closeted was influenced by their perceptions of the level of sexism, heterosexism, and homonegativity within their particular setting and context, as well as reflecting their familial relationships over time. However, focus group members who were grandparents believed that asking family members (e.g., grandchildren) to accept their sexuality may pose too great a challenge because, traditionally, grandparents are expected to guard and protect their grandchildren from both real and imagined foes (King, Russell, & Elder, 1998). Lesbian grandmothers did not disclose their sexual orientation specifically because they believed that they were protecting their grandchildren from real foes (e.g., social stigma and discrimination) and they also believed that they were protecting themselves from possibly being estranged from their families. For those focus group members who were not "out" to family members, there was the belief that this prevented emotionally close relationships. Conversely, for those members who were "out" and accepted by their families, familial support was viewed as being extremely important for their sense of happiness and wellbeing.

The needs and concerns of the focus group participants frequently varied based on whether they were "out" and the level of comfort with their sexual orientation identity. This level of disclosure touched on all of the areas identified; their level of comfort with their sexual orientation identity was often a reflection of the social stigma that they had experienced. For example, one focus group member indicated that the negative societal messages about homosexuality that she experienced made her hesitant about disclosing her sexual orientation. She indicated that "perhaps this is due to a small part of me believing these negative messages."

The finding that focus group members' ability to maintain supportive relationships with family and friends were becoming more challenging as they aged was particularly informative and it was evident that this required additional investigation. Likewise, the finding that they experienced social stigma and systematic discrimination based on their sexual orientation *and* age was extremely important, yet it gave little indication of the prevalence of social stigma and systematic discrimination in the general LGBT older adult community. Finally, the finding that the intensity of need and concern within the seven major areas of importance varied for "out" focus group members when compared to those who had not disclosed their sexual orientation to family, friends, colleagues, or practitioners required additional investigation. Therefore, it was evident that a comprehensive needs assessment instrument was necessary, which would build on the findings from the focus group discussions and would address the seven areas identified in the focus group discussions (medical/health care, legal, institutional/housing, spiritual, family, mental health, and social) with a special emphasis on disclosure status.

LGBT NEEDS ASSESSMENT SURVEY

The findings from the analysis of the focus group participants' comments led to the development and distribution of an extensive self-report survey instrument that specifically included both forced-response ($n = 104$) and open-ended questions ($n = 32$) on the areas identified in the focus group discussions. The specific number of questions a respondent would answer varied based on personal factors such as age, physical/mental health status, level of community involvement, life experiences, and so on. For example, one question asked whether counseling services were ever used. If the respondent answered yes, they were then asked to provide information for why they sought counseling (i.e., sadness, anxiety, addiction, etc.). Another question asked respondents to indicate whether their legal needs/concerns were being adequately met. If the answer was "no," they were asked to describe the unmet needs or services that they would like to receive.

Collectively, the LGBT Elders Needs Assessment Scale provides a way in which to assess the perceived needs in seven life areas (medical/health care, legal, institutional/housing, spiritual, family, mental health, social), perceptions of unmet needs, and levels of involvement and satisfaction with service providers. For example, within the medical/health care category, respondents are asked to (a) rate their current overall health using a Likert scale ranging from 1 (*very poor*) to 7 (*excellent*), (b) identify current major chronic health conditions (i.e., arthritis, diabetes, HIV/AIDS, etc.), (c) identify areas in which assistance is needed (i.e., dressing, shopping, bathing, etc.), (d) indicate number of physician/medical doctor visits in the past year and indicate the number of prescribed medications that are taken on a daily basis. In addition to these forced response health related questions, respondents are also asked to identify their current health insurance coverage and the type of health services/programs that they received within the past month. Open-ended questions asked respondents to identify any unmet medical needs for which they are not receiving care and to list the type of services that they would like to receive. To assess the impact of heterosexism on LGBT older adults' access to affirmative health services, there were questions included in the survey that asked respondents to indicate whether they were "out" or open about their sexual orientation/identity/lifestyle to their doctor, therapist, or case manager. Respondents who indicated that they were not "out" to any of the aforementioned providers were asked to list the main reasons for their lack of disclosure. Another forced-response question asked respondents to answer "yes" or "no" to the following: "Do you believe there are any positive benefits to disclosing your sexual orientation to your service provider or anyone in the health care field, now or in the future?" Respondents who answered "yes" were asked to list those benefits. Respondents were also asked if they would prefer to visit a clinic, health care provider, or counselor that openly promoted services to LGBT elders. These responses can be categorized and analyzed along with respondents' sociodemographic background (e.g., age, gender, socioeconomic status, race, ethnicity, religion, relationship status, work history, education, and housing).

Because it was apparent from the focus group discussions that the needs and concerns of the participants were different based on whether they were "out" and the level of comfort with their sexual orientation, a modified Burdon's Openness Scale (Davis, 1998) was also included in the needs assessment survey. This scale has been used to measure participants' level of "outness" and their level of comfort with their sexual orientation identification and was modified for a middle-aged and older adult population. Respondents are asked to rate themselves on a scale of 1 (*never*) to 5 (*always*) regarding how out or open they are about their sexual identity/orientation. Sample questions include, "I attempt to hide my homosexuality from members of my family and friends," "I let my straight friends know that I am LGBT," and "I am open with my medical or service provider about my sexual orientation."

The LGBT Elders Needs Assessment Scale is currently in the field being completed by participants. The length of time in which this survey has been available has been considerable, but it has been the goal to be able to obtain the voices of numerous LGBT older adults from diverse groups. One of the most challenging tasks in conducting any research with LGBT older adults is actually being able to locate this population in order to recruit their participation for specific research projects. Therefore, a variety of methods have been used to recruit potential participants and assistance from identified colleagues and "agents" has been key. Agents are individuals known to this researcher who have access to potential respondents. These agents are often LGBT older adult themselves or are staff at organizations/agencies that provides programs and services to older adults. Academic colleagues have been instrumental in all aspects of the research activities, but especially in the recruitment of respondents. Because recruitment of participants from more than one geographical location was the goal, academic colleagues from numerous locations were instrumental in being able to reach this goal.

Participants who belonged to older gay men and lesbian friendship networks (e.g., Lavender Triangle and Gay and Gray), support groups (e.g., PrimeTimers), or religious organizations (e.g., Dignity and Lutherans Concerned) were also recruited by this researcher, identified colleagues, and "agents." We were able to gain entry into the established LGBT older adult community through personal acquaintances and assistance from advocacy groups in a variety of geographical locations. Local mental health counselors who advertise in local LGBT business guides were also contacted and used to identify potential participants. In addition to recruiting participants from LGBT community organizations, it was also imperative to recruit LGBT participants who may not be members of LGBT community organizations. Therefore, multipurpose senior centers, assisted living facilities, continuing care retirement centers, and area agencies on aging were approached by the researchers to post flyers that asked for research participants. It is important to note that agencies/organizations within the aging network of providers, as well as LGBT advocacy groups were very supportive of these research activities and the Executive Director of one particular senior center specifically requested assistance in planning programs/services that would meet the needs of LGBT elders within her county. The most successful method of recruitment, however, was "word of mouth" or "snowballing" (a common approach used in the general model of qualitative methods; Patton, 2002). With both of these methods, participants who had been members of a focus group or who had completed surveys informed their LGBT friends of the research project. These individuals then contacted the researchers and requested surveys or volunteered to participate in subsequent research. This speaks highly of the willingness of many LGBT older adults to have their voices heard by participating in research and the need for these issues to be given a platform.

To protect the confidentiality of the participants, the identity of those who complete the survey instrument will remain anonymous. As previously indicated, participants will be able to obtain the survey at a variety of sites (e.g., multipurpose senior centers, LGBT organizations, religious organizations, and health care agencies) and participants are provided with preaddressed, prepaid envelopes to return their completed surveys.

Because the analysis of the data from the LGBT Elders Needs Assessment Scale is ongoing, only preliminary results can be reported. To date, approximately 2,000 questionnaires have been distributed and slightly more than one-half have been returned ($n = 1,150$). Respondents range in age from 64 to 88 years of age ($M = 73$), and 83% live in an urban setting. There are 736 women who identified their sexual orientation as lesbian or bisexual (64%) and 414 gay men (36%). Ninety-one percent of the participants are Caucasian, 8% African American, and less than 2% are Latino or Latina. It is obvious from the preliminary results that greater emphasis must be placed on reaching a more racially/ethnically diverse sample that also includes transgender older adults. Because the vast majority of respondents (73%) indicated that they are out and comfortable with their self-identified LGB label, greater emphasis must also be placed on reaching LGBT older adults who have not disclosed their sexual orientation. The finding that 73% of the respondents were out is similar to findings from the *MetLife Study of Lesbian, Gay, Bisexual, and Transgender Baby Boomers* (MetLife, 2010) that found that 75% of gay men and 60% of lesbian respondents were out to most others. However, similar to the MetLife national survey, LGBT older adults who completed the needs assessment reported variations in which they were and were not open with in regard to their sexual orientation.

Although the majority of respondents indicated that they are out and comfortable with their self-identified LGB label, the responses to the questions that assessed their perceptions and satisfaction with services and programs for older adults revealed that slightly more than 53% (n = 615) were dissatisfied with the services because these services did not meet their unique needs as LGB older adults. When asked what factors affect their use of traditional aging network programs/services (e.g., congregate meals at senior centers, home health care, and social work/case management services), 32% (n = 368) responded "discrimination or fear of discrimination." Twenty-two percent of LGB respondents also indicated that they faced discrimination when seeking housing at "traditional" retirement communities, and 42% reported negative experiences with the health care system related to their sexual orientation. Most respondents (83%) indicated their overwhelming interest in participating in social groups exclusively for LGBT older adults, living in a community designated for LGBT older adults, and visiting clinics/health care providers that openly promote services to LGBT elders. These results not only speak of respondents' desire for LGBT affirming programs and services, but also suggest that LGBT older adults are reliant on nontraditional sources of support (i.e., friends or family of choice) because of their unfavorable experiences with traditional aging network programs/services. However, their ability to create strong networks of friends or family of choice was also identified by participants as being one of their primary strengths and an advantage of being LGB, similar to findings of the 2006 MetLife study.

It is anticipated that a full analysis of the responses for the LGBT Elders Needs Assessment Scale will bring new awareness to the issues, concerns, and needs facing LGBT older adults, as well as their level of involvement and satisfaction with agencies and organizations that provide services to the older adult population. However, the review of early returned surveys led to an unanticipated, but welcomed new line of research. As previously indicated, the initial needs assessment survey included a variety of demographic questions that included asking respondents about their relationship histories (e.g., not in a relationship, in a same-sex relationship, in a heterosexual marriage, widowed from a heterosexual relationship) and whether they had children and the ages of children. A number of lesbians indicated on their surveys that a question concerning the number of grandchildren that they had was not included in the survey. Although this was not an intended omission, it was an indication of this researcher's lack of awareness and perhaps a reflection of internalized cultural messages concerning LGBT persons. Historically, the terms *lesbian mother, gay father, lesbian grandmother,* and *gay grandfather* have been viewed as contradiction in terms (Bigner, 1996, 2000; Clunis & Green, 2003; Orel & Fruhauf, 2006) because homosexuality was viewed as being inconsistent with the ability to procreate and, as a result, become a parent and grandparent. These lesbian women clearly informed this researcher that their specific needs and concerns of being a lesbian grandmother were not being addressed in this specific needs assessment and perhaps elsewhere in their lives. Their concerns also mirrored the comments made by the two lesbian grandmothers who participated in the previously described focus groups with LGB older adults. Therefore, subsequent printings of the LGBT Elders Needs Assessment Survey included a question concerning whether respondents were grandparents. The experiences of LGB grandparents became a special area of focus of the unmet and diverse needs of LGBT older adults. Preliminary results are described as follows.

INDIVIDUAL INTERVIEWS WITH LGB GRANDPARENTS

I undertook a pilot project to investigate the significance of grandmothers' sexual orientation on the grandparent–grandchild relationship. It was not my goal to focus exclusively on women, but it was my intention to conduct individual interviews with the lesbian grandmothers who had completed the needs assessment survey and who had specifically indicated that they would be willing to discuss their experiences and provide their feedback to the assessment instrument. Most important, the primary goal of this project was to obtain a deeper appreciation, understanding, and awareness of the grandparent–grandchild relationship when grandmothers defined their sexual orientation as lesbian or bisexual.

Although numerous studies have explored the grandparent–grandchild relationship and the variables that affect this "vital" (Kornhaber & Woodward, 1981), "enduring" (Bengston, 2001), and "significant" (Kivett, 1991) relationship, one variable that had not been explored was the centrality of sexual orientation on the grandparent–grandchild relationship. Because previous research on grandparenting and grandparenthood has not included sexual orientation as a research variable, accurate estimations of the number of LGBT grandparents are not available. However, it has been estimated that there are over ten million children currently living with three million LGB parents in the United States (Mercier & Harold, 2003). Because 94% of older adults with children will become grandparents (Smith & Drew, 2001), applying this statistic to the estimated three million LGB parents, a conservative range of one to two million LGB individuals are (or will soon become) grandparents. In addition, with the increase in same-sex couples adopting children, finding surrogate mothers to bear children, and becoming pregnant through artificial insemination (Flaks, Ficher, Masterpsqua, & Joseph, 1995; Johnson & O'Connor, 2002; C. J. Patterson, 1995), it is likely that the current and future aging LGB population will experience grandparenthood in greater numbers than previous LGB cohorts. In addition, the number of LGB grandparents may even be larger, given the previously mentioned unknown numbers of individuals who do not live openly LGB lives. As the number of LGBT individuals becoming grandparents increase, it is imperative that the grandparent–grandchild relationship within the context of LGBT families be understood and appreciated.

Orel (2004b, 2006b) and Orel and Fruhauf (2006) were the first to specifically explore the effects of sexual orientation on the grandparent–grandchild relationship by using the life course perspective as a guide. The life course perspective on relationships between grandparents and grandchildren focuses on roles embedded within the social/historical life course, providing for the necessary temporal quality and examination of individual differences to relationships in later-life families. The trajectory of the relationships is built on the experiences within the specific relationships and broader familial relationships in the past. The historical influence of the family of origin and earlier family experiences provide the background from which the current role and relationship evolve. This perspective allows for the understanding of the linked lives of intergenerational relationships and the diversity and heterogeneity within intergenerational relationships. The direction and degree of change within relationships illustrate the multiple pathways that intergenerational relationships follow across time. Applying the life course perspective to lesbian and bisexual (LB) grandmothers, it was assumed that the grandparent–grandchild relationship is embedded within the context of the grandmother's individual choices across the lifespan (e.g., decisions to disclose one's homosexuality), the structural contexts within which these decisions are made (e.g., level of homophobia within a culture), and the transitions that grandmothers experienced (e.g., previous heterosexual marriages and divorce).

As previously mentioned, the initial participants for this research were lesbian grandmothers who indicated on their LGBT Needs Assessment Survey that a question concerning the number of grandchildren that they had was not included in the survey. These lesbian grandmothers also provided unsolicited contact information and indicated and that they would be willing to "talk about being a lesbian grandmother." Additional participants for the face-to-face individual interviews were recruited using a modified snowball sampling method (Patton, 1990). To date, the participants in the research that explored LB grandmothers' perceptions of their relationships with their grandchildren included 31 lesbian grandmothers and 7 bisexual grandmothers who ranged in age from 43 to 75 ($M = 59.9$). Thirty-two grandmothers identified themselves as Caucasian, with five identifying themselves as African American and one as "other." The majority of LB grandmothers ($n = 33$) were previously involved in heterosexual marriages. Thirty of those relationships ended in divorce, with the remaining three ending with the death of the husband. At the time of the interview, all but five of the grandmothers were in partnered relationships (ranging from 1 week–21 years). Collectively, the participants had 78 grandchildren ranging in age from 9 months to 38 years, and 26 great-grandchildren ranging in age from 6 months to 20 years. The LB grandmothers were living in the Midwest (Ohio and Michigan) at the time of the interview. Each interview was approximately 90 to 120 min in length, and all interviews were audiotaped. Although an interview guide was used as an outline of topics of potential theoretical importance (e.g., the relationship between their lesbian or bisexual identity and their identity as grandmothers), participants were encouraged to freely discuss their experiences as a lesbian or bisexual grandmother.

In recognition of the gendered experience of grandparenting, it was apparent that research that would focus on the experiences of gay men as grandfathers was needed. Therefore, in tandem with the research focusing on LB grandmothers, semi-structured individual interviews with gay grandfathers were being conducted. Fruhauf, Orel, and Jenkins (2009) specifically examined the experiences of gay grandfathers' coming-out processes to their grandchildren. Participants in this study included eleven grandfathers living in Texas and ranging in age from 40 to 79 years old. All grandfathers identified themselves as Caucasian and six had earned a college degree (2 bachelor's degrees, 2 master's degrees, 1 juris doctoral degree, and 1 doctoral degree). All but four of the grandfathers were currently working at the time of the interview. All grandfathers were in a heterosexual relationship prior to coming out and reported that their marriage ended in divorce. After their divorce, the participants lived openly as gay men. Eight grandfathers were partnered (ranging from 3 months–17 years) at the time of the interview. All grandfathers reported having children (ranging from 2–4 children) and reported having a range of two to seven grandchildren. Grandfathers reported their grandchildren (a total of 45 grandchildren) ranged in age from 6 months to 30 years.

Given the exploratory nature of the research with LGB grandparents, a general model of qualitative procedures (i.e., a method used to discover and interpret the perspectives of individuals studied) and data analysis (Merriam, 1998) was used to explain and interpret the centrality of sexual orientation on the grandparent–grandchild relationship and the coming out process of LGB grandparents to their grandchildren. Qualitative methods are well suited for understanding the complexity of family issues (Daly, 1992) and for understanding close relationships (Allen & Walker, 2000). Various techniques (i.e., triangulation, peer examination, recognition of our research bias, and thick description) were used as a means to insure trustworthiness and credibility. Themes emerged from the data that represented recurring patterns and relationships between and among the narratives provided by the participants. LGB grandparents' perceptions of the grandparent–grandchild relationship consisted of three themes. These three themes were (a) the formation of a LGB grandparent identity, (b) the centrality of sexual orientation in the LGB grandparent–grandchild relationship, and (c) the impact of externalized or internalized homonegativity on the LGB grandparent–grandchild relationship. I have addressed these themes in previous research (Orel, 2004b, 2006b); in the section that follows, I focus on the second theme, and its constituents, elaborating on the discussion of disclosure and its consequences.

Throughout all of the face-to-face, semi-structured, in-depth interviews with LGB grandparents, their descriptions of their relationships with their grandchildren were always placed within the context of their on-going relationship with their adult children (Fruhauf, Orel, & Jenkins, 2009; Orel, 2004b, 2006b; Orel & Fruhauf, 2006). LGB grandparents who had strong, intimate relationships with their adult children were more likely to have close relationships with their grandchildren. Adult children also determined the amount of access that LGB grandparents, or in some cases their partners, would have with their grandchildren. Therefore, adult children mediated the development of the relationship between LGB grandparents and their grandchildren, and the *mediating role of parents in the grandparent–grandchild relationship when grandparents are LGB* was a category under the overarching theme labeled the *centrality of sexual orientation on the grandparent–grandchild relationship.* This finding concurs with previous literature on the grandparent–grandchild relationship that stressed that the grandparent–grandchild relationship should be conceptualized as an indirect one with parents as intermediaries (Matthews & Sprey, 1985). Parents are the gatekeepers to the grandparent–grandchild relationship and they can facilitate or discourage the development of an emotionally intimate relationship between the grandparents and grandchildren (Whitbeck, Hoyt, & Huck, 1993). This long-standing finding that parents are the intermediaries of the grandparent–grandchild relationship was amplified for LGB grandparents.

It was also evident that adult children's acceptance of the grandparents' sexual orientation determined LGB grandparents' opportunities to grandparent and that adult children's attitudes toward homosexuality influenced the direction of the mediating effect (i.e., facilitating or discouraging) on the grandparent–grandchild relationship. The LGB grandparents were aware of the impact that their sexual orientation had on their relationships with their adult children and subsequently their grandchildren. It is important to note that four of the 16 LB grandmothers were completely secretive about their sexual orientation, with neither their adult children nor grandchildren being aware of their self-identification as lesbian or bisexual women. For those LB grandmothers who did not disclose their sexual orientation to their adult children or grandchildren, they expressed profound fear and anxiety concerning what would happen to their relationship with their grandchildren if their sexual orientation was known. The LB grandmothers' level of concern was specifically related to their assumptions that their adult children would not be able to accept their sexual orientation and would then prevent them from seeing their grandchildren. This speaks not only to the influence of the parent in the grandparent–grandchild relationship, but how parents can also influence or inhibit disclosure.

Levels of honest discourse between generations was a subcategory that emerged under *the mediating role of parents in the grandparent–grandchild relationship when grandparents are LGB* category. The decision-making process surrounding whether to "come out" to adult children and grandchildren, and subsequently the ability to either remain secretive or disclose their sexual orientation to adult children and grandchildren was a significant event for all LGB grandparents (echoing the findings noted in the studies reported earlier). However, the actual process of coming out to adult children and grandchildren varied amongst the LGB grandparents. The initial research on LB grandmothers indicated that adult children not only influenced the formation and maintenance of the grandmother–grandchild relationship, but they played a profound and significant role in the coming out process of LB grandmothers (Orel, 2006b; Orel & Fruhauf, 2006; S. Patterson, 2005). It is important to note that all LB grandmothers indicated that their sexual orientation *per se* was not significant in regard to their ability to assume the grandmother role and their subsequent relationships with their grandchildren. Rather, the significance of their sexual orientation was related to their ability to have an open and honest relationship with adult children and grandchildren. Honesty and openness was severely compromised when LB grandmothers were fearful of disclosing an important personal dimension of their identity: their sexual orientation. It is important to note that this fear was created and fueled by the heterosexist and homophobic context in which the LB grandmother–grandchild relationship was embedded (Orel, 2006b; Orel & Fruhauf, 2006; S. Patterson, 2005).

The gender of adult children (parents) also played a significant role in the coming out process of LB grandparents (Orel, 2006b; Orel & Fruhauf, 2006). Among adult children, it was women (mothers) who were more likely than men (fathers) to facilitate understanding of grandmothers' homosexuality with their children. A primary reason that women facilitated LB grandmothers' disclosure to their grandchildren was that generally it was women who were more likely to be aware of their mothers' sexual orientation. This finding is similar to general LGBT research that found that female family members are more likely to be aware of LGBT kin and more likely to be the recipient of disclosure than male family members (Ben-Ari, 1995; Savin-Williams & Ream, 2003).

Gay grandfathers took many different approaches to disclosing their sexual orientation to their grandchildren, but all gay grandfathers indicated that adult children played a profound role in the coming out process, along the lines of the mediating role of adult children as described earlier. Another consistent finding in the available LGB grandparent research is the emphasis that LGB grandparents give to being able to disclose their sexual orientation to their grandchildren. For LGB grandparents, disclosing their sexual orientation was psychologically salient. LGB grandparents who disclosed to adult children and grandchildren indicated that they were seeking emotional support, understanding, acceptance, and unconditional love. Because it is the common expectation that grandparents are the providers of unconditional love and emotional support to their grandchildren, when LGB grandparents do seek this unconditional love and emotional support when they disclose their sexual orientation, this can be viewed by adult children and grandchildren as going against familial expectations and roles. Accepting an LGB grandparent's sexual orientation was difficult for some family members, as reported by LGB grandparents, but the opportunity to be open and honest was viewed as psychologically important for LGB grandparents. LGB grandparents reported that disclosure provided a level of sincere honesty that only intensified the emotional closeness that they experience with their grandchildren. It was also very evident that LGB grandparents' decision to disclose was influenced by the history of family relationships and the expectations of current roles and relationships.

Collectively, it was apparent from the individual interviews that LGB grandparents are a diverse group of individuals. However, the research also revealed the following predominant themes: (a) Managing disclosure about sexual orientation is the primary issue for all LGB grandparents, (b) the decision to disclose is based on a variety of factors (i.e., disclosure status with adult child, age/developmental level of grandchildren, requests from adult children to disclose or remain secretive, beliefs that grandchildren would be protected if they remain closeted, desire to increase partner's status as co-grandparent, and social conditions), (c) adult children play a profound role in the coming out process of LGB grandparents, and (d) the decision to come out takes into consideration the level of sexism, heterosexism, and homonegativity within a particular culture/context. These findings also illustrate that for LGB grandparents, "coming out" or disclosing one's sexual orientation is a life-long process with varying passages and multiple results. This confirms the importance of including measures of "outness," measures of level of comfort with sexual orientation, as well as including measures of the varying and dynamic social and familial roles played by LGBT older adults on any needs assessment instrument.

Based on these findings from the face-to-face interviews with LGB grandparents, a survey has been developed that will be distributed nationally to obtain a more comprehensive understanding of the grandparent–grandchild relationship when grandparents self-identify as being LGBT. Because research is especially needed to investigate the experiences of transgendered grandparents and co-grandparents (e.g., non-biological grandparents) this survey will specifically include questions that are inclusive for transgendered grandparents and co-grandparents.

DISCUSSION AND RECOMMENDATIONS

The results of the reported qualitative and quantitative research contribute to our knowledge and understanding of the unique needs and concerns facing LGBT older adults and suggest several implications for future research. The most noteworthy implication is the recognition that the needs and concerns of LGBT older adults be addressed across multiple domains, rather than in isolation. For example, many LGBT persons are also members of other groups that face substantial discrimination. These groups have had to navigate multiple instances of discrimination based on race, ethnicity, language, degree of physical ability, geographic location, etc. Future research needs to focus on understanding the implications of differences in race, ethnicity, cultural environments, socioeconomic status, and age among LGBT older adults utilizing the intersectionality perspective that examines multiple identities and the ways in which they interact (Crenshaw, 1989; Institute of Medicine, 2011). It is also imperative to recognize that an LGBT older adult does not belong to one homogenous group within the LGBT acronym (Mabey, 2011). Therefore, any investigation of the needs and concerns among LGBT older adults must take into consideration multiple attributes of the population and the interlocking systems of vulnerability and need that result in the cumulative effects of a lifetime of discrimination and stigma:

> While most Americans face challenges as they age, LGBT elders have the added burden of a lifetime of stigma; familial relationships that lack recognition under the law; and unequal treatment under laws, programs and services designed to support and protect older Americans. Further, the lack of financial security, good health and health care, and social and community support is a fearful reality for a disproportionate number of LGBT older adults. (SAGE, 2010, p. 1)

What was clearly evident from the research with LGB older adults is that their greatest obstacle is the level of homophobia and heterosexism within the culture and perhaps within their own families. However, all research participants identified advantages, and these advantages evolved from their ability to survive (and thrive) within a heterosexist culture. The research participants also believed that being an LGB person better prepared them for aging (e.g., greater self-reliance, increased attention to legal/financial matters, and the ability to create strong support systems). The ability of, and necessity for LGBT individuals to cope with discrimination and overcome adversity across the lifespan has been identified as being important in preparing LGBT persons for the demands of aging within an ageist society. This finding has been reported by numerous researchers who have concluded that LGBT older adults have increased crisis competence, or mastery of stigma when faced with the challenges associated with aging (Cahill et al., 2000; de

Vries, 2011; Kimmel, 1978; MetLife, 2010, Quam & Whitford, 1993; Shippy, Cantor, & Brennan, 2004). Specifically, the coming out process enables LGBT individuals to develop a competency for dealing with other crises throughout the lifespan (Heaphy, 2007; Kimmel, 2002; McFarland & Sanders, 2003; MetLife, 2006; Morrow, 2001; Quam, 1993).

It was evident from the interviews with LGB grandparents that the process of disclosing one's LGB identity to their adult children and grandchildren was considered a key event in the development of their emotionally close familial relationships. However, all LGB grandparents indicated that coming out, or revealing their sexual orientation was a lifelong process with varying passages and multiple results—for themselves and perhaps for changing cultural attitudes. Many LGB grandparents believed that if they could be open about their sexual orientation with their grandchildren, then perhaps their grandchildren would become advocates for LGBT persons and, thus, reduce heterosexism in their schools or communities. LGB grandparents, who had disclosed their sexual orientation, voiced their desires to be recognized as a grandparent who just happens to be LGB. However, they also wanted the saliency of their sexual orientation to be acknowledged by social, health, and educational practitioners.

Because practitioners typically assume that grandparents are heterosexual, practitioners working with LGBT grandparents may overlook the saliency of grandparents' sexual orientation on the grandparent–grandchild relationship. Practitioners must avoid the use of heterosexist language and heteronormative assumptions and listen for subtle messages to learn about an older adult's sexual identity and orientation. Otherwise, practitioners who assume heterosexuality will overlook the unique challenges, issues, and concerns of LGBT grandparents. Unfortunately, for most LGBT grandparents the "invisibility" of their status as a grandparent exacerbates their general sense of invisibility as an LGBT older adult. LGBT grandparents (and their partners) must receive the social support and recognition that is naturally granted to heterosexual grandparents within all cultures. Practitioners must also recognize that because LGBT grandparents have developed creative and resourceful ways to function within a heterosexist culture as LGBT *persons,* LGBT grandparents can provide creative and flexible definitions of grandparenting and grandparenthood.

Because there has been a complete "invisibility" of transgender grandparents within both the gerontological and LGBT literature (Cook-Daniels, 2006; MetLife, 2011), the perceptions and experiences of transgender grandparents must be explored. The literature on grandparenting tends to highlight that being a grandparent is a gendered familial role and that grandparenting holds different expectations for behaviors and responsibilities for men and women (Mann, 2007; Stelle, Fruhauf, Orel, & Landry-Meyer, 2010; Thomas, 1994). However, an inconsistency exists between the assumption and findings that the sex of the grandparental generation is an important factor to consider and how little transgender grandparents and their experiences within the family have been explored. In this way, transgendered grandparents remain invisible as the subject of research. Likewise, the exploration of the ways in which gender *and* sexual orientation influences grandparenting remains largely unexplored. With the unprecedented growth in the general older adult population and subsequently the LGBT older adult population, it is without question that LGBT grandparents will increase in number. The specific needs and concerns of LGBT grandparents must be researched and policy and practice focusing on these intergenerational relationships is especially needed. Future planned research will investigate (a) how LGBT grandparents conceptualize their identity knowing that they are both members of a marginalized sexual minority and, yet, hold a highly regarded and respected position as a grandparent, (b) the differences in experiences and roles of LGBT grandparents if they are the biological grandparent, co-grandparent, step grandparent, or social grandparent, and (c) the psychological wellbeing of LGBT grandparents. An extensive self-report instrument for LGBT grandparents has been developed and it will be nationally distributed.

Collectively, the research reported here suggests that additional research is needed to fully comprehend the unique issues facing LGBT older adults so that programs and services that have been designed to support and protect the general older adult population would also address the specific needs and concerns of LGBT older adults. Examining the needs and concerns of LGBT grandparents, and LGBT older adults in general provides numerous opportunities for practitioners to reflect on the assumptions that are often evident in the current provision of services and programs for the general older adult population. Tragically, research has shown that there continues to be heterosexism within aging service providers and this tends to marginalize LGBT older adults with discriminatory policies and stigmatization (Cahill et al., 2000). Confronting the heterosexism that exists within traditional aging service providers will require collaborative endeavors between the aging network and the LGBT community. With additional research and developments such as the recent establishment of the National Resource Center on LGBT Aging, appropriate, adequate, and affirming services for LGBT older adults may become a reality.

REFERENCES

Administration on Aging. (2010). *A profile of older Americans: 2010*. Washington, DC: U.S. Department of Health and Human Services.

Allen, K. R., & Walker, A. J. (2000). Qualitative research. In C. Hendrick & S. Hendrick (Eds.), *Close relationships: A sourcebook* (pp. 19–30). Thousand Oaks, CA: Sage.

Barranti, C., & Cohen, H. (2000). Lesbian and gay elders: An invisible minority. In R. Schneider, N. Kropt, & A. Kisor (Eds.), *Gerontological social work: Knowledge, service settings, and special populations* (2nd ed., pp. 343–367). Belmont, CA: Wadsworth.

Ben-Ari, A. (1995). The discovery that an offspring is gay: Parents', gay men's, and lesbian's perspectives. *Journal of Homosexuality, 30*, 89–111.

Bengston, V. (2001). Beyond the nuclear family: The increasing importance of multigenerational bonds. *Journal of Marriage & the Family, 63*, 1–16.

Bigner, J. (1996). Working with gay fathers: Developmental, postdivorce parenting, and therapeutic issues. In J. Laird & R. J. Green (Eds.), *Lesbians and gays in couples and families: A handbook for therapists* (pp. 370–403). San Francisco, CA: Jossey-Bass.

Bigner, J. (2000). Gay and lesbian families. In W. Nichols, M. Pace-Nichols, D. Becvar, & A. Napier (Eds.), *Handbook of family development and intervention* (pp. 279–298). Hoboken, NJ: Wiley.

Cahill, S., South, K., & Spade, J. (2000). *Outing age: Public policy issues affecting gay, lesbian, bisexual, and transgendered elders*. New York, NY: Policy Institute of the National Gay and Lesbian Task Force.

Carlat, D. J., Camargo, C. A., & Herzog, D. B. (1997). Eating disorders in males: A report on 135 patients. *American Journal of Psychiatry, 154*, 1127–1132.

Carpenter, C. (2003). Sexual orientation and body weight: Evidence from multiple surveys. *Gender Issues, 21*(3), 60–74.

Clunis, D., & Green, G. (2003). *The lesbian parenting book: A guide to creating families and raising children*. New York, NY: Seal.

Cochran, S. (2001). Emerging issues in research on lesbians' and gay men's mental health: Does sexual orientation really matter? *American Psychologist, 56*, 931–947.

Cochran, S., & Mays, V. (2000). Lifetime prevalence of suicide symptoms and affective disorders among men reporting same-sex sexual partners: Results using BHANES III. American *Journal of Public Health, 90*, 573–977.

Cochran, S., & Mays, V. (2006). Estimating prevalence of mental and substance-using disorders among lesbians and gay men from existing national health data. In A. Omoto & H. Kurtzman (Eds.), *Sexual orientation and mental health* (pp. 143–165). Washington, DC: American Psychological Association.

Cochran, S., & Mays, V. (2009). Burden of psychiatric morbidity among lesbian, gay, and bisexual individuals in the California Quality of Life Survey. *Journal of Abnormal Psychology, 118*, 647–658.

Cochran, S., Mays, V., Bowen, S., Gage, D., Bybee, S., Roberts, R., . . .White, J. (2001). Cancer-related risk indicators and preventive screening behaviors among lesbians and bisexual women. *American Journal of Public Health, 91*, 591–597.

Cook-Daniels, L. (2006). Trans aging. In D. Kimmel, T. Rose, & S. David (Eds.), *Research and clinical perspectives on lesbian, gay, bisexual, and transgender aging* (pp. 20–52). New York, NY: Columbia University Press.

Crenshaw, K. (1989). *Demarginalizing the intersection of race and sex: A Black feminist critique of antidiscrimination doctrine, feminist theory, and antiracist politics*. Chicago, IL: University of Chicago Legal Forum.

Daling, J. R., Weiss, N. S., Hislop, T. G., Maden, C., Coates, R. J., Sherman, K. J., . . . Corey, L. (1987). Sexual practices, sexually transmitted diseases, and the incidence of anal cancer. *New England Journal of Medicine, 317*, 973–977.

Daly, K. (1992). The fit between qualitative research and characteristics of families. In J. Gilgun, K. Daly, & G. Handel (Eds.), *Qualitative methods in family research* (pp. 3–11). Newbury Park, CA: Sage.

D'Augelli, A. R., & Patterson, C. (1996). *Lesbian, gay, and bisexual identities over the lifespan.* New York, NY: Oxford University Press.

Davis, C. (1998). *Service needs, availability and satisfaction among lesbians age 40+.* (Master Thesis). Retrieved from http://content.lib.utah.edu/utils/getfile/collection/ehsl-GerInt/id/19/filename/65.pdf

Dean, L., Meyer, I. H., Robinson, K., Sell, R. L., Sember, R., Silenzio, V., . . . Tierney, R. (2000). Lesbian, gay, bisexual, and transgender health: Findings and concerns. *Journal Gay Lesbian Medical Association, 4*, 102–151.

Denenberg, R. (1995). Report on lesbian health. *Women Health Issues, 5*, 181–191.

Deputy, N., & Boehmer, U. (2010). Determinants of body weight among men of different sexual orientation. *Prevention Medicine, 51*, 129–131.

de Vries, B. (2011, July/August). LGBT aging comes of age and holds lessons for all elders. *Aging Today.* Retrieved from http://www.asaging.org/blog/lgbt-aging-comes-age-and-holds-lessons-all-elders

Diamanti, A., Schuster, M., & Lever, J. (2000). Receipt of preventative health care services by lesbians. *American Journal of Preventive Medicine, 19*, 141–148.

Diamanti, A., Wold, C., Spritzer, K., & Gelberg, L. (2000). Health behaviors, health status, and access to and use of health care: A population-based study of lesbian, bisexual, and heterosexual women. *Archives of Family Medicine, 9*, 141–148.

Dibble, S. L., Vanoni, J. M., & Miaskowski, C. (1997). Women's attitudes toward breast cancer screening procedures: Differences by ethnicity. *Women's Health Issues, 7*, 47–54.

Dorfman, R., Walter, K., Burke, P., Hardin, I., Karanik, T., Raphael, J., & Silverstein, E. (1995). Old, sad, and alone: The myth of the aging homosexual. *Journal of Gerontological Social Work, 24*(1/2), 29–44.

DuRant, R. H., Krowchuk, D. P., & Sinal, S. H. (1998). Victimization, use of violence, and drug use at school among male adolescents who engage in same-sex sexual behavior. *Journal of Pediatrics, 133*, 113–118.

Fergusson, D. M., Horwood, J., & Beautrais, A. L. (1999). Is sexual orientation related to mental health problems and suicidality in young people? *Archives of General Psychiatry, 56*, 876–880.

Ferrini, A., & Ferrini, R. (2000). *Health in the later years* (3rd ed.). New York, NY: McGraw-Hill.

Flaks, D., Ficher, I., Masterpsqua, F., & Joseph, G. (1995). Lesbians choosing motherhood: A comparative study of lesbian and heterosexual parents and their children. *Developmental Psychology, 37*, 105–114.

Fruhauf, C., Orel, N., & Jenkins, D. (2009). Grandfathers' perceptions of their adult children's influence on their coming out process to grandchildren. *Journal of Gay, Lesbian, Bisexual, and Transgender Family Studies, 5*, 99–118.

Gates, W. (2011). *How many people are lesbian, gay, bisexual, and transgender?* Los Angeles, CA: Williams Institute, UCLA School of Law.

Gay and Lesbian Medical Association. (2001). *Healthy People 2010: Companion document for lesbian, gay, bisexual, and transgender (LGBT) health*. San Francisco, CA: Author.

Glaser, B. G., & Strauss, A. L. (1967). *The discovery of grounded theory: Strategies for qualitative research*. Chicago, IL: Aldine.

Grant, J., Koskovick, G., Frazer, S., & Bjerk, S. (2010). *Outing Age 2010: Public policy issues affecting lesbian, gay, bisexual, and transgender elders*. Washington, DC: National Gay and Lesbian Task Force Policy Institute.

Heaphy, B. (2007). Sexualities, gender, and ageing. *Current Sociology, 55*, 193–210.

Herdt, G., & de Vries, B. (2004). Introduction. In G. Herdt & B. de Vries (Eds.), *Gay and lesbian aging: Research and future directions* (pp. xi–xxii). New York, NY: Springer.

Herek, G. M. (2009). Hate crimes and stigma-related experiences among sexual minority adults in the United States: Prevalence estimates from a national probability sample. *Journal of Interpersonal Violence, 24*, 54–74.

Hunter, S. (2005). *Midlife and older LGBT adults: Knowledge and affirmative practice for social services*. Binghamton, NY: Hawthorn.

Hunter, S. (2007). *Coming out and disclosures: LGBT persons across the life span*. Binghamton, NY: Haworth.

Institute of Medicine. (1998). *Leading health indicators for Healthy People 2010*. Washington, DC: National Academies Press.

Institute of Medicine. (1999). *Lesbian health: Current assessment and directions for the future*. Washington, DC: National Academies Press.

Institute of Medicine. (2011). *The health of lesbian, gay, bisexual, and transgender people: Building a foundation for better understanding*. Washington, DC: National Academies Press.

Johnson, S., & O'Connor, E. (2002). *The gay baby boom: The psychology of gay parenthood*. New York, NY: New York University Press.

Kimmel, D. (1978). Adult development and aging: A gay perspective. *Journal of Social Issues, 34*, 113–130.

Kimmel, D. (2002). Aging and sexual orientation. In B. E. Jones & M. J. Hill (Eds.), *Mental health issues in lesbian, gay, bisexual, and transgender communities* (pp. 17–36). Washington, DC: American Psychiatric Association.

Kimmel, D., Rose, T., Orel, N., & Greene, B. (2006). Historical context for research on lesbian, gay, bisexual, and transgender aging. In D. Kimmel, T. Rose, & S. David (Eds.), *Research and clinical perspectives on lesbian, gay, bisexual, and transgender aging* (pp. 1–26). New York, NY: Columbia University Press.

King, V., Russell, S. T., & Elder, G. H. (1998). Grandparenting in family systems: An ecological perspective. In M. E. Szinovacz (Ed.), *Handbook on grandparenthood* (pp. 53–69). Westport, CT: Greenwood.

Kinsey, A. C., Pomeroy, W. B., & Martin, C. E. (1948). *Sexual behavior in the human male*. Philadelphia, PA: Saunders.

Kivett, V. (1991). The grandparent–grandchild connection. *Marriage and Family Review, 16*, 267–290.

Koblin, B., Hessol, N., Zauber, A., Taylor, P., Buchbinder, S., Katz, M., & Stevens, C. (1996). Increased incidence of cancer among homosexual men, New York

City and San Francisco, 1978–1990. *American Journal of Epidemiology, 144,* 916–923.

Kochman, A. (1997). Gay and lesbian elderly: Historical overview and implications for social work practice. *Journal of Gay and Lesbian Social Services, 6*(1), 1–10.

Koh, A. (2000). Use of preventive health behaviors by lesbian, bisexual, and heterosexual women: Questionnaire survey. *Western Journal of Medicine, 172,* 379–384.

Koh, A., & Ross, L. (2006). Mental health issues: A comparison of lesbian, bisexual, and heterosexual women. *Journal of Homosexuality, 51*(1), 33–57.

Kornhaber, A., & Woodward, K. L. (1981). *Grandparents/grandchildren: The vital connection.* Garden City, NY: Anchor.

Lincoln, Y. S., & Guba, E. G. (1985). *Naturalistic inquiry.* Beverly Hills, CA: Sage.

Mabey, J. E. (2011). Counseling older adults in LGBT communities. *Professional Counselor, 1*(1), 57–62.

Mann, R. (2007). Out of the shadows?: Grandfatherhood, age and masculinities. *Journal of Aging Studies, 21,* 281–291.

Matthews, S. H., & Sprey, J. (1985). Adolescents' relationships with grandparents: An empirical contribution to conceptual clarification. *Journal of Gerontology, 40,* 621–626.

Mayer, K. H., Bradford, J. B., Makadon, H. J., Stall, R., Goldhammer, M. S., & Landers, S. (2008). Sexual and gender minority health: What we know and what needs to be done. *American Journal of Public Health, 98,* 989–995.

Maykut, P., & Morehouse, R. (1994). *Beginning qualitative research: A philosophic and practical guide.* London, England: Falmer.

McFarland, P. L., & Sanders, S. (2003). A pilot study about the needs of older gays and lesbians: What social workers need to know. *Journal of Gerontological Social Work, 40*(3), 67–80.

Mercier, L., & Harold, R. (2003). A feminist approach to exploring the intersection of individuals, families, and communities: An illustration focusing on lesbian mother research. *Journal of Human Behavior in the Social Environment, 7*(3/4), 79–95.

Merriam, S. (1998). *Qualitative research and case study applications in education.* San Francisco, CA: Jossey-Bass.

MetLife. (2006). *Out and aging: The MetLife study of lesbian and gay baby boomers.* Westport, CT: MetLife Mature Market Institute.

MetLife. (2010). *Still out, still aging: The MetLife study of lesbian, gay, bisexual, and transgender baby boomers.* Westport, CT: MetLife Mature Market Institute.

Meyer, I., & Northridge, M. (2007). *The health of sexual minorities: Public health perspectives on lesbian, gay, bisexual, and transgender populations.* New York, NY: Springer.

Morgan, D. L. (1997). *Focus groups as qualitative research* (2nd ed.). Thousand Oaks, CA: Sage.

Morrow, D. F. (2001). Older gays and lesbians: Surviving a generation of hate and violence. *Journal of Gay & Lesbian Social Services, 13*(1/2), 151–169.

National Gay and Lesbian Task Force Policy Institute. (1999). *Aging initiative.* Washington, DC: Author.

Orel, N. (2004a). Gay, lesbian, bisexual elders: Expressed needs and concerns across focus groups. *Journal of Gerontological Social Work, 43*(2/3), 57–77.

Orel, N. (2004b, November). *Lesbian and bisexual women as grandmothers: The centrality of sexual orientation on the grandparent–grandchild relationship.* Paper presented at the 57th annual scientific meeting of the Gerontological Society of America, Washington, DC.

Orel, N. (2006a). Community needs assessment: Documenting the need for affirmative services for gay, lesbian, and bisexual elders. In D. Kimmel, T. Rose, & S. David (Eds.), *Research and clinical perspectives on lesbian, gay, bisexual, and transgender aging* (pp. 321–346). New York, NY: Columbia University Press.

Orel, N. (2006b). Lesbian and bisexual women as grandparents: The centrality of sexual orientation on the grandparent–grandchild relationship. In D. Kimmel, T. Rose, & S. David (Eds.), *Research and clinical perspectives on lesbian, gay, bisexual, and transgender aging* (pp. 248–274). New York, NY: Columbia University Press.

Orel, N., & Fruhauf, C. (2006). Lesbian and bisexual grandmothers' perceptions of the grandparent–grandchild relationship. *Journal of Gay, Lesbian, Bisexual, and Transgender Family Studies, 2*(1), 43–70.

Patterson, C. J. (1995). Sexual orientation and human development: An overview. *Developmental Psychology, 31*, 3–11.

Patterson, S. (2005). Better one's own path: The experiences of lesbian grandmothers in Canada. *Canadian Woman Studies, 24*, 118–122.

Patton, M. Q. (1990). *Qualitative evaluation and research methods* (2nd Edition). Newbury Park, CA: Sage.

Patton, M. Q. (2002). *Qualitative research & evaluation methods* (3rd ed.). Thousand Oaks, CA: Sage.

Ponce, N., Cochran, S., Pizer, J., & Mays, V. (2010). The effects of unequal access to health insurance for same-sex couples in California. *Health Affairs, 29*(8), 1539–1548.

Quam, J. K. (1993). Gay and lesbian aging. *SIECUS Report, 21*(5), 10–12.

Quam, J. K., & Whitford, G. (1992). Adaptation and age-related expectations of older gay and lesbian adults. *Gerontologist, 32*, 367–374.

Richardson, D., & Seidman, S. (2002). *Handbook of lesbian and gay studies.* New York, NY: Sage.

Robertson, P., & Schachter, J. (1981). Failure to identify venereal disease in a lesbian population. *Sexually Transmitted Diseases, 8*(2), 75–76.

Savin-Williams, R. C., & Ream, G. (2003). Sex variations in the disclosure to parents of same-sex attractions. *Journal of Family Psychology, 17*, 429–438.

Seidman, S. (2002). *Beyond the closet: The transformation of gay and lesbian life.* New York, NY: Routledge.

Services and Advocacy for Gay, Lesbian, and Transgender Elders (SAGE). (2010). *Improving the lives of LGBT older adults.* Denver, CO: LGBT Movement Advancement Project.

Services and Advocacy for GLBT Elders. (2010, April). Understanding and meeting the needs of LGBT elders. *SAGE News.* Retrieved from https://www.sageusa.org/newsevents/release.cfm?ID=59&print=1

Shippy, R., Cantor, M., & Brennan, M. (2004). Social networks of aging gay men. *Journal of Men's Studies, 13*(1), 107–120.

Skinner, W., & Otis, M. (1996). Drug and alcohol use among lesbian and gay people in a southern U.S. sample: Epidemiological, comparative, and methodological findings from the Trilogy Project. *Journal of Homosexuality, 30*(3), 59–92.

Smith, P., & Drew, L. (2002). Grandparenthood. In M. Bernstein (Ed.), *Handbook of parenting, Vol. 3: Being and becoming a parent* (2nd ed., pp. 141–172). Mahwah, NJ: Erlbaum.

Stall, R. D., Greenwood, G. L., Acree, M., Paul, J., & Coates, T. J. (1999). Cigarette smoking among gay and bisexual men. *American Journal of Public Health, 89,* 1875–1878.

Stall, R., & Wiley, J. (1988). A comparison of alcohol and drug use patterns of homosexual and heterosexual men: The San Francisco Men's Health Study. *Drug and Alcohol Dependence, 22,* 63–73.

Stelle, C., Fruhauf, C., Orel, N., & Landry-Meyer, L. (2010). Grandparenting in the 21st century: Issues of diversity in grandparent–grandchild relationships. *Journal of Gerontological Social Work, 53,* 682–701.

Stewart, D. W., & Shamdasani, P. N. (1990). *Focus groups: Theory and practice. Applied Social Research Methods Series (Vol. 20).* Newbury Park, CA: Sage.

Tang, H., Greenwood, G., Cowling, D., Lloyd, J., Roeseler, A., & Bal, D. (2004). Cigarette smoking among lesbians, gays, and bisexuals: How serious a problem? *Cancer Causes and Control, 15,* 797–803.

Thomas, J. L. (1994). Older men as fathers and grandfathers. In F. Thompson (Ed.), *Older men's lives* (pp. 197–217). Thousand Oaks, CA: Sage.

U.S. Census Bureau. (2000). *Statistical abstract of the United States.* Washington, DC: Government Printing Office.

Whitbeck, L. B., Hoyt, D. R., & Huck, S. M. (1993). Family relationship history, contemporary parent–grandparent relationship quality, and the grandparent–grandchild relationship. *Journal of Marriage & the Family, 55,* 1025–1035.

Zaritsky, E., & Dibble, S. (2010). Risk factors for reproductive and breast cancers among older lesbians. *Journal of Women's Health, 19*(1), 125–131.

Friends, Family, and Caregiving Among Midlife and Older Lesbian, Gay, Bisexual, and Transgender Adults

CATHERINE F. CROGHAN, MS, MPH, RN
Croghan Consulting, Roseville, Minnesota, USA

RAJEAN P. MOONE, PhD
Greater Twin Cities United Way, Minneapolis, Minnesota, USA

ANDREA M. OLSON, PhD
Psychology Department, St. Catherine University, St. Paul, Minnesota, USA

The study examines the frequency and nature of the informal caregiving experience for midlife and older lesbian, gay, bisexual, or transgender (LGBT) adults. Responses from a Twin Cities Metropolitan Area LGBT aging needs assessment survey were analyzed for social supports, current caregiving activity and availability of a caregiver. The majority of respondents identified a primary caregiver who was not a legal relation; and compared to the general population were (a) less likely to have traditional sources of caregiver support and (b) more likely to be serving as a caregiver and caring for someone to whom they were not legally related. Implications of the findings for enhancing resources to more fully support the 10% of caregivers that are caring for non-kin are discussed.

Although only 5% of older adults reside in a skilled nursing facility or nursing home (Hillier & Barrow, 2010), placement in a nursing home remains one of the primary fears of the American public. Having a family caregiver is a key indicator for remaining in your home and in your community (Miller & Weissert, 2000; Spillman & Long, 2009). Family caregiving, in contrast to formal caregiving, is the unpaid assistance of any relative, partner, friend or neighbor who provides a broad range of assistance for an older adult or an adult with chronic or disabling conditions (AARP, 2011). In 2009 an estimated 61.6 million U.S. family caregivers provided care valued at $450 billion. This unpaid care is a central feature of the overall United States long-term social services and health care plan for maintaining the fast-growing population of older adults in the community. As a result, there is considerable interest in development of policies, programs and services that will sustain caregivers in their critical roles. What does this mean for lesbian, gay, bisexual, or transgender (LGBT) caregivers?

FAMILY FACTORS

Family caregiving for older adults is primarily a female activity, with 85% done by wives, and adult daughters and daughter-in-laws (National Alliance for Caregiving & AARP, 2011) and usually follows a hierarchical pattern with assistance sought first from spouses followed by adult children, other relatives and finally neighbors and friends (Shanas, 1980). This order reflects traditional family patterns and is less appropriate for LGBT older adults (Barker, Herdt, & de Vries, 2006) who are less likely to have children and partners than the larger population (Adelman, Gurevich, de Vries, & Blando, 2006; Beeler, Rawls, Herdt, & Cohler, 1999; Cantor, Brennan, & Shippy, 2004; Croghan, Mertens, Yoakam, & Edwards, 2003; de Vries, 2006; Fredriksen, 1999; Grossman, d'Augelli, & Hershberger, 2000; MetLife, 2010) and who cannot marry a same-sex partner in most States (National Gay and Lesbian Task Force, 2012). Further, some LGBT adults lack the support of extended biological families due to the stresses or estrangement associated with the coming out process (Cantor et al., 2004; de Vries & Hoctel, 2006; Witten, 2009).

Due to a lack of biological and legal family to provide support, many older LGBT individuals will rely on friends to sustain them in the community. A common feature of LGBT culture is the "chosen family" which comprises people with whom you feel close and consider family even though they are not biologically or legally related to you (MetLife, 2010). The MetLife study of LGBT baby boomers found 64% reported having a family of choice.

SERVICE PROVIDER READINESS TO WORK WITH LGBT CLIENTS

These families of choice often form the caregiving networks that support LGBT older adults in the community (de Vries, 2011). However, LGBT care recipients and caregivers may find a service provider network that is ill prepared to meet their needs. A 2010 national survey of Area Agencies on Aging (AAAs; Knochel, Croghan, Moone, & Quam, 2012) found < 13% of AAAs conducted outreach to the LGBT community, < 8% reported LGBT targeted services and about one-third had staff trained in LGBT aging issues. Sixty percent did not believe there was a need to address issues specific to LGBT people, and while approximately three-fourths believed LGBT people would be welcomed by local senior service providers, the balance did not believe they would be welcomed or were unsure of a positive welcome. A national survey of nursing home social service directors found only 24% had received at least 1 hr of training about homophobia in the previous five years (Bell, Bern-Klug, Kramer, & Saunders, 2010). At major national conferences of aging service providers, opportunities for education on LGBT aging has also been minimal (Moone & Cagle, 2011). Multiple local and regional studies suggest only a minority of providers are prepared to work with LGBT clients (Knochel, Quam, & Croghan, 2011; Logie et al., 2008; Willingin, Salvador, & Kanan, 2006).

NON-KIN CAREGIVING

The overall lack of service provider readiness to work with LGBT clients may be exacerbated by the high rate of non-kin caregiving in the LGBT community. Approximately ten percent of U.S. caregiving is provided by someone not legally related to the care receiver (Barker, 2002). This rate is considerably higher for the LGBT community due to non-heteronormative family structures. Fredriksen-Goldsen et al. (2011) reported 27% of LGBT adults 50 and older were serving as caregivers. This included 35% providing care to a partner or spouse, 32% caring for a friend and 7% caring for some other non-related persons such as a neighbor. The MetLife (2010) study of LGBT baby boomers found 21% serving as caregivers of whom 34% caring for a partner or spouse, 21% caring for a friend and 6% caring for a neighbor or someone else.

Caregiving can have a number of negative effects on the caregiver including their financial position, retirement security, social relations, careers, and physical and emotional health (AARP, 2011). The associated high levels of caregiver stress result in poor outcomes for both the caregiver and care receiver and are strong predictors of nursing home placement (Spillman & Long, 2009).

Non-kin caregivers and their care recipients experience added stress due to the limited support resources available to them. Although the National Family Caregiver Support Act provides for assistance to all primary caregiver regardless of relationship, many federal and state laws and policies are reserved for caregivers caring for someone to whom they are legally related. These include coverage under the Family Medical Leave Act, equivalent Medicaid spend-downs, Social Security benefits and bereavement leave (Fredriksen-Goldsen & Hoy-Ellis, 2007). Legal documents such as durable powers of attorney for health care and wills need to be executed to ensure that wishes of non-kin caregivers and care receivers are honored.

FEAR OF ACCESSING SERVICES

In addition to interacting with a service provider network that may not be ready to work with them, LGBT caregivers may be reluctant to seek services or disclose their LGBT identities when seeking services due to fear of receiving poor quality services or being denied services. Multiple surveys in Australia, Canada and the United States suggest LGBT adults do not believe they will be welcomed or receive high quality services when accessing aging services if their sexual orientation or gender identity were known (Brotman, Ryan, & Cormier, 2003; Croghan et al., 2003; de Vries, 2006; Hughes, 2009). This anticipation of discrimination may result from personal experiences or those shared by their personal network (Brotman et al., 2007). In addition to LGBT clients not being confident of a welcoming service provider environment, non-LGBT specific survey respondents have indicated they too are unsure that LGBT individuals will receive appropriate care. Jackson, Johnson, and Roberts (2008) reported the majority of both heterosexual and LGB survey participants believed long-term care residents and staff would discriminate based on sexual orientation. A 2007 survey of AAA service providers in Minneapolis–St. Paul found 38% believed lesbian and gay older adults would not be welcomed at local senior centers (Knochel et al., 2011).

RELUCTANCE TO DISCLOSE

Delivery of quality services to LGBT caregivers may also be hindered by the reluctance of LGBT clients to disclose their sexual orientation or gender identity due to fear of discrimination when seeking social and health services. de Vries's (2006) review of multiple U.S. and Canadian LGBT community surveys showed up to 24% did not disclose their sexual orientation to service providers, or rarely discussed it. The Caring and Aging with Pride Project (Fredriksen-Goldsen et al., 2011) found 11% of LGBT respondents had not told their primary physician about their sexual orientation or gender identity. A national survey of transgender individuals found 28% of respondents had postponed health care due to fears of discrimination (Grant, Mottet, & Tanis, 2010). Cantor et al. (2004) studying LGBT caregivers in New York City report 50% did not disclose sexual orientation to service providers.

Disclosure of sexual orientation to a medical provider has been shown to be positively linked to regular health care use (Steele, Tinmouth, & Lu, 2006). The failure to disclose makes LGBT people invisible to service providers (Brotman et al., 2003; Clark, Landers, Linde, & Sperber, 2001; Fredriksen-Goldsen et al., 2011; Jackson et al., 2008) and, therefore, limits their ability to deliver appropriate services and medical care specific to the client.

PURPOSE AND RATIONALE

Even with previous studies detailing trends in LGBT caregiving, much is still unknown about the diversity of the LGBT caregiving experience. This study sheds additional light on the frequency and nature of caregiving within the LGBT community at midlife and older ages. The data used in this study were derived from a 2012 Twin Cities Metropolitan Statistical Area (MSA; U.S. Census Bureau, 2012) LGBT aging needs assessment survey that was intended to generate information for use in local planning (Croghan, Moone, & Olson, 2012). Responses from individuals 48 years old (the youngest baby boomers) and older were included in this study.

METHOD

Participants

A total of 792 people responded to the survey and ranged in age from 18 to 85 years old. Of those, 242 (31%) were younger than 48 and were, thus, excluded for the purposes of this study. Of the remaining 551 respondents, 56 participants were excluded if they reported a zip code outside of the Twin Cities MSA, or if they reported they were both cisgender[1] and heterosexual. The final sample consisted of 495 participants.

Three in ten respondents (29.7%; $n = 147$) were 48 to 54 years old, 45.5% ($n = 225$) were between the ages of 55 and 64 years old, 20.4% ($n = 101$) were 65 to 74 years of age, and 4.4% ($n = 22$) were 75 and older (see Table 1).

Nine percent ($n = 45$) were bisexual, 46.7% ($n = 231$) were lesbians, 38.7% ($n = 191$) were gay men, and 5.3% ($n = 26$) were queer/other. Nine in 10 (90.1%) were cisgender, including 247 women and 199 men. Approximately 10% were transgender, including 31 women, 16 men, and 2 non-male/female identified individuals.

The sample was predominantly White, non-Latino (93.2%), and most participants had a Bachelor of Arts/Bachelor of Science or more formal education (80.8%). Less than one-third were retired (29%). Less than 1 in 10 (7.5%) reported household incomes under $20,000, and more than one-fourth (26.5%) reported a household income of $100,000 or more.

TABLE 1 Sample Demographics

Variable	n	%
Gender identity		
Transgender woman	31	6.3
Transgender man	16	3.2
Transgender other	2	<1
Cisgender woman	247	49.9
Cisgender man	199	40.2
Sexual orientation		
Gay man	191	38.6
Lesbian	231	46.7
Bisexual woman	26	5.2
Bisexual man	19	3.8
Queer/other	26	5.3
Heterosexual	2	<1
Age		
48–54 years	147	29.7
55–64 years	225	45.5
65–74 years	101	20.4
>74 years	22	4.4
Relationship status		
Single	186	39.0
Partnered/married	283	59.5
Widowed	7	1.5
Education		
<High school	2	<1
High school diploma/general equivalency diploma	37	7.7
Some college	53	11.1
Bachelor's degree	137	28.6
Advanced degree	250	52.2
Race/ethnicity		
African American	17	3.9
Asian/Pacific Islander	<5	<1
Latino	<5	<1
Native American	<5	<1
White, non-Latino	410	93.2
Other not listed	7	1.6
Retired	137	29.0
Annual household income		
<$20,000	33	7.5
$20,000–$39,999	76	17.3
$40,000–$59,000	87	19.8
$60,000–$79,000	77	17.5
$80,000–$99,000	50	11.4
$100,000+	117	26.5

Survey

Survey questions were developed using a similar survey administered in 2002 on the needs of aging LGBT people (Croghan et al., 2003). Recent national and regional studies also informed the development of the survey and provided comparison data, including *Still Out, Still Aging: The MetLife study of LGBT baby boomers* (MetLife, 2010), *Aging and Health Report: Disparities and resilience among LGBT adults* (Fredriksen-Goldsen et al., 2011), and the *Survey of Older Minnesotans* (Minnesota Board on Aging, 2005).

The survey contained 45 items. Twenty-eight of the items were demographic and background questions, and 17 questions related to aging, including questions about family and community connections and caregiving.

There were six items covering social supports and connections. They included questions about relationship status (not partnered/single, partnered/married, or widowed), living arrangements (alone, with a partner or spouse, or with others), whether the participant had children (yes, no), family of origin acceptance of the person's life as an LGBT person, whether the participant had enough close friends (yes or no), and whether the participant had a chosen family (yes or no).

There were four items specifically about caregiving. They asked if the participant was currently providing care for another person (yes or no) and, if so, who that person was; and whether the participant had someone who would take care of them (yes or no) and, if so, who their own primary caregiver would be.

Procedure

Twenty-one community partners (20 LGBT organizations and 1 LGBT aging advocate) sent recruitment e-mails with an embedded electronic survey link to their organization members and associates. These combined contact lists reached approximately 5,900 addresses. Researchers did not have access to the individual lists, but assumed there was considerable overlap and that some individuals received more than one recruitment e-mail. To enable participation by individuals without computer or Internet access, the electronic survey distribution was supplemented with a limited distribution of a paper version. A total of 198 paper surveys, including a stamped and addressed return envelope, were distributed by four partners who reported having constituents that were not reached by e-mail and other electronic communications. Upon return, completed paper survey responses were entered into the online database. Thirty-six of the 198 responded for a response rate of 18%. Instructions in both the electronic and paper surveys included a request that recipients complete the survey only once. However, there was no way to screen survey responses for potential duplicate submissions.

Initially, community partners were asked to forward the invitation e-mail with survey link three times (initial recruitment and 2 reminder e-mails) to their constituents during the four-week survey period, from mid-February to mid-March, 2012. Five potential partners pointed out that they wished to participate but could not make multiple contacts. These organizations forwarded the invitations at least once during the four-week survey period.

Data Analysis

The primary focus of this article is on three predictor variables (age, sexual orientation, and gender identity) and eight criteria variables (i.e., relationship status, living arrangements, children, family acceptance, having enough close friends, chosen family, caregiving status, and having an available caregiver for oneself). By including both sexual orientation and gender identity as predictor variables, the analysis avoids conflating these concepts. However, because each respondent has a reported age, sexual orientation and gender identity, there will be apparent overlap in samples used in the analyses. For example, reporting on relationship status for gay men and cisgender men will include many of the same subjects in both results (i.e., cisgender men who are also gay).

Three main types of analyses were conducted: descriptive statistics were calculated (such as count [n value]), mean, standard deviation, and percentage), nonparametric statistics (i.e., chi-square analyses) and standardized residual scores (SRS) to follow up on the nonparametric test results. When a chi-square analysis yields significant results, SRS may be used to identify the cells that contribute most to the chi-square value. An SRS is the difference between the expected value and observed value, standardized into a z score. This standardized score can then be compared to a critical z score that corresponds to a desired level of significance. For a significance level of $p = .05$, the corresponding critical z score is 1.96. If the absolute value of the SRS in a cell is > 1.96 then the actual frequency differs significantly from the expected frequency, and thus differs significantly from what would be expected by chance. This follow-up analysis allows us to identify the cells that contribute most to the overall chi-square.

RESULTS

Relationship Status

Most respondents were partnered/married (59.5%; $n = 283$), 186 participants (39.1%) reported they were single, and 7 (1.5%) indicated they were widowed (see Table 2). Relationship status was not related to age but was related to sexual orientation. The first chi-square analysis conducted for relationship status and sexual orientation indicated there were five cells with expected values < 5, which was 33.3% of the cells. The criterion used for this research was that no more than 20% of cells in a chi-square analysis were allowed to have expected values < 5. In those cases, categories were either collapsed or removed and data were reanalyzed. In this case, there were seven participants who were widowed. Their data were removed, and results showed a significant chi-square with no cells having expected values < 5, $\chi^2(4, N = 467) = 22.80$, $p < .01$. Significantly fewer gay men were partnered/married than expected by chance (47.0%; $n = 85$; SRS = − 2.3)

TABLE 2 Social Supports (Living Arrangement, Relationship Status, and Children) by Age, Sexual Orientation and Gender Identity

Variable	Relationship Status				Living Arrangement				Children		
	Single %	Partner %	Widow %	Total n	Alone %	Partner/Spouse %	Other %	Total n	Yes %	No %	Total n
Total	39.1	59.5	1.5	476	39.5	50.7	9.8	479	35.4	64.6	480
Age	39.1	59.5	1.5	476	39.5	50.7	9.8	479	35.4	64.6	480[a]
48–54	38.7	60.6	0.7	142	36.2	48.2	15.6	141	31.5	68.5	143
55–64	36.1	62.1	1.8	219	37.9	54.3	7.8	219	31.1	68.9	219
65–74	44.2	54.7	1.1	95	43.9	49.0	7.1	98	47.4	52.6	97
75+	50.0	45.0	5.0	20	57.1	38.1	4.8	21	52.4	47.6	21
Sexual orientation	39.0	59.5	1.5	474[b]	39.6	50.7	9.6	477[c]	35.4	64.6	478[d]
Gay man	51.6	45.7	2.7	186	50.3	39.6	10.2	187	22.8	77.2	189
Lesbian	30.2	68.9	0.9	225	32.9	58.8	8.3	228	38.1	61.9	226
Bisexual woman	29.2	70.8	0.0	24	33.3	58.3	8.3	24	66.7	33.3	24
Bisexual man	33.3	66.7	0.0	18	29.4	58.8	11.8	17	77.8	22.2	18
Queer/other	38.1	61.9	0.0	21	33.3	47.6	19.0	21	47.6	52.4	21
Gender identity	39.0	59.5	1.5	474[e]	39.4	50.7	9.9	477[f]	35.4	64.6	478[g]
Transgender woman	30.8	69.2	0.0	26	23.1	69.2	7.7	26	69.2	30.8	26
Transgender man	56.3	43.8	0.0	16	50.0	37.5	12.5	16	37.5	62.5	16
Cisgender woman	30.5	68.6	0.8	239	33.5	56.6	9.9	242	38.3	61.7	240
Cisgender man	49.2	48.2	2.6	193	48.2	42.0	9.8	193	27.0	73.0	196

[a] $\chi^2(3, N = 480) = 11.56$, $p < .01$. [b] $\chi^2(4, N = 467) = 22.80$, $p < .01$ (for this analysis, those who were widowed were excluded: $n = 7$; when they were included, five cells in the chi-square analysis had expected values < 5, which was 33.3% of the cells; when those who were widowed were excluded, there were zero cells with expected values < 5). [c] $\chi^2(8, N = 477) = 19.38$, $p < .05$. [d] $\chi^2(4, N = 478) = 39.71$, $p < .01$. [e] $\chi^2(3, N = 467) = 19.77$, $p < .01$ (for this analysis, those who were widowed were excluded: $n = 7$; when they were widowed were excluded, four cells in the chi-square analysis had expected values < 5, which was 33.3% of the cells; when those who were widowed were excluded, there were zero cells with expected values < 5). [f] $\chi^2(6, N = 477) = 15.27$, $p < .05$. [g] $\chi^2(3, N = 478) = 19.95$, $p < .01$.

and significantly more gay men were single (53.0%; $n = 96$; SRS = 2.9). Significantly fewer lesbians were single than expected by chance (30.5%; $n = 68$; SRS = −2.2).

Relationship status was also related to gender identity. Significantly fewer cisgender women indicated they were single compared to what would be expected by chance (30.8%; $n = 73$; SRS = −2.2) and significantly more cisgender men were single than expected by chance (50.5%; $n = 95$; SRS = 2.4), $\chi^2(3, N = 476) = 19.77, p < .01$.

Living Arrangement

Slightly over one-half (50.7%; $n = 243$) lived in a household with a partner or spouse, 39.5% ($n = 189$) lived alone, and 9.8% ($n = 47$) had some other living arrangement including living with roommates, other relatives (not a partner or spouse), or group setting (see Table 2).

The rate of living alone increased with age with 36.2% ($n = 51$) of those 48 to 54 years old living alone, increasing to 57.1% ($n = 12$) for 75 years and older. The rate of living alone was highest among transgender men at 50.0% ($n = 8$), followed by 48.2% ($n = 93$) of cisgender men. One-half of gay men lived alone (50.3%; $n = 94$), which was significantly greater than what would be expected by chance, $\chi^2(8, N = 477) = 19.38, p < .05$ (SRS = 2.3).

The highest rates of living with a partner or spouse were observed in transgender women (69.2%; $n = 18$) followed by lesbians (58.8%; $n = 134$), bisexual men (58.8%; $n = 10$), bisexual women (58.3%; $n = 14$), and cisgender women (56.62%; $n = 137$). Only 39.6% ($n = 74$) of gay men lived with a partner or spouse, which was significantly less than what would be expected by chance, $\chi^2(8, N = 477) = 19.38, p < .05$ (SRS = −2.1).

Children

Slightly more than one-third (35.4%; $n = 170$) reported having children (see Table 2). The percentage of those 65 and older who had children was 48.3% ($n = 57$), which was significantly greater than what would be expected by chance when age categories were collapsed, $\chi^2(2, N = 480) = 11.37, p < .01$ (SRS = 2.4). This dropped to 31% ($n = 113$) for respondents under 65 years of age.

Bisexual men (77.8%; $n = 14$), transgender women (69.2%; $n = 18$), and bisexual women (66.7%; $n = 16$) reported the highest rates of having children when looking at the variables of age, sexual orientations, and gender identities. Each of those percentages was greater than what would be expected by chance: For sexual orientation, $\chi^2(4, N = 478) = 39.71, p < .01$ (SRS bisexual men = 3.0, SRS bisexual women = 2.6); for gender identity, $\chi^2(3, N = 478) = 19.95, p < .01$ (SRS transgender women = 2.9).

The percentage of gay men who had children (22.8%; $n = 43$) and cisgender men who had children (27.0%; $n = 53$) were significantly less than what would be expected by chance (SRS gay men $= -2.9$; SRS cisgender men $= -2.0$).

Acceptance by Family of Origin

Almost two-thirds (63.7%; $n = 284$) reported their family of origin to be extremely or very accepting of their life as an LGBT person (see Table 3). However, 10.1% ($n = 45$) reported their families to be not at all accepting or not very accepting. The pattern of acceptance by family of origin was significantly related to sexual orientation, $\chi^2(4, N = 445) = 19.88, p < .01$. For this chi-square analysis, those who indicated they were bisexual women, bisexual men or queer or other orientation were combined into one group. (When they were separate, 5 cells in the chi-square analysis had expected values < 5, which was 33.3% of the cells. When bisexual women, bisexual men, and other orientation were combined into one group, there were 0 cells with expected values < 5.) As a combined group, significantly fewer bisexual women, bisexual men and those who indicated other orientation reported their family of origin to be extremely or very accepting of their life as an LGBT person (38.5%; $n = 20$; SRS $= -2.3$) compared to what was expected by chance, and significantly more reported their family of origin to be not at all accepting or not very accepting (23.1%; $n = 12$; SRS $= 2.9$) compared to what was expected by chance.

Close Friends

The majority of respondents reported having enough close friends (65.1%; $n = 296$; see Table 3). There were no significant differences across age groups. The pattern of having enough close friends was significantly related to sexual orientation, $\chi^2(4, N = 453) = 9.98, p < .05$; and gender identity, $\chi^2(3, N = 453) = 10.12, p < .05$. Relatively more bisexual women reported having enough close friends (86.4%; $n = 19$).

Chosen Family

Three-fourths (75.6%; $n = 340$) reported having a chosen family, defined as a group of people to whom you are emotionally close and consider "family," although you are not biologically or legally related (see Table 3). Rates were fairly similar for age, sexual orientation and gender identity groups with the exception of relatively fewer bisexual men who reported having a family of choice (50%; $n = 8$).

TABLE 3 Social Supports (Family Acceptance, Enough Close Friends, and Chosen Family) by Age, Sexual Orientation, and Gender Identity

Variable	Family Acceptance				Enough Close Friends			Chosen Family		
	Not At All/ Not Very %	Somewhat %	Very/Total %	Total	Yes %	No %	Total	Yes %	No %	Total
Total	10.1	26.2	63.7	446	65.1	34.9	455	75.6	24.4	450
Age	10.1	26.2	63.7	446	65.1	34.9	455	75.6	24.4	450
48–54	9.2	28.5	62.3	130	67.7	32.3	130	73.8	26.2	130
55–64	9.2	29.1	61.7	206	64.6	35.4	209	75.0	25.0	208
65–74	11.0	18.7	70.3	91	62.5	37.5	96	78.5	21.5	93
75+	21.1	15.8	63.2	19	65.0	35.0	20	78.9	21.1	19
Sexual orientation	10.1	26.1	63.8	445[a]	65.1	34.9	453[b]	75.4	24.6	448
Gay man	8.4	26.4	65.2	178	64.8	35.2	179	75.3	24.7	178
Lesbian	8.4	22.8	68.8	215	64.8	35.2	219	77.2	22.8	215
Bisexual woman	14.3	38.1	47.6	21	86.4	13.6	22	77.3	22.7	22
Bisexual man	40.0	26.7	33.3	15	37.5	62.3	16	50.0	50.0	16
Queer/other	18.8	50.0	31.3	16	70.6	29.4	17	76.5	23.5	17
Gender identity	9.9	26.3	63.8	445	65.1	34.9	453[c]	75.4	24.6	448
Transgender woman	13.6	22.7	63.6	22	65.2	34.8	23	69.6	30.4	23
Transgender man	13.3	40.0	46.7	15	26.7	73.3	15	73.3	26.7	15
Cisgender woman	8.8	25.7	65.5	226	66.7	33.3	231	77.5	22.5	227
Cisgender man	10.4	26.4	63.2	182	66.3	33.7	184	73.8	26.2	183

[a] $\chi^2(4, N = 445) = 19.88, p < .01$ (for this analysis, those who indicated they were bisexual women, bisexual men, or other orientation were combined into one group; when they were separate, five cells in the chi-square analysis had expected values < 5, which was 33.3% of the cells; when bisexual women, bisexual men, and other orientation were combined into one group, there were zero cells with expected values < 5). [b] $\chi^2(4, N = 453) = 9.98, p < .05$. [c] $\chi^2(3, N = 453) = 10.12, p < .05$.

Caregiving

Just over one in five were currently serving as caregivers (22.2%; $n =$ 101) and there were few differences across age groups (see Table 4). The pattern of caregiving was significantly related to gender identity, $\chi^2(2, N =$ $452) = 8.41, p < .05$. For this chi-square analysis, those women and men who indicated they were transgender were combined into one group because the original chi-square showed that more than 20% of cells had an expected value < 5. When transgender women and transgender men were combined into one group, there were 0 cells with expected values < 5. Results showed that two-thirds of caregivers (66.3%) were women.

The pattern of caregiving was also significantly related to sexual orientation, $\chi^2(3, N = 452) = 11.01, p < .05$. For this chi-square analysis, those who indicated they were bisexual women or bisexual men were combined into one group. When bisexual women and bisexual men were combined into one group, there was 1 cell with an expected value < 5 (12.5%). Significantly more bisexual adults in this sample were caregivers than what was expected by chance (SRS = 2.2). Bisexual women were caregivers at twice the rate of bisexual men.

For groups that had a sufficient number of people indicating they were caregivers (i.e., > 10), bisexual women (50%; $n = 11$) had the highest rate of caregiving, followed by cisgender women (25.7%; $n =$ 59) and lesbians (24.4%; $n = 53$). Cisgender men (15.7%; $n = 29$) and gay men (16.1%; $n =$ 29) reported the lowest rates of caregiving.

Caregivers most frequently reported caring for a parent or parent-in-law (40.6%; $n = 41$), followed by 30.7% ($n = 31$) caring for a friend or neighbor, 18.8% ($n = 19$) caring for a spouse or partner, 11.9% ($n = 12$) caring for a brother/sister or other relative, 5.0% ($n = 5$) caring for a child or child-in-law, and 2.0% ($n = 2$) caring for a grandchild (see Table 4). (Respondents could select more than 1 person.)

Available Caregiver

More than three-fourths (78.3%; $n = 357$) reported having someone to take care of them if they were sick or unable to care for themselves (see Table 5). The highest rate was reported by those 75 and older (85.0%; $n = 17$). The lowest rates of available caregivers were reported by queer or other sexual orientations (76.5%; $n = 13$), cisgender men (74.7%; $n = 139$), gay men (72.9%; $n = 132$), and transgender men (60.0%; $n = 9$).

Of the 354 people who responded to the item asking who they would consider their own primary caregiver, 70.1% ($n = 248$) indicated a partner or spouse (see Table 5). Approximately 13.8% ($n = 49$) indicated a friend or neighbor, 5.6% ($n = 20$) indicated a child or child-in-law, 5.6% ($n = 20$) indicated other relative, 3.4% ($n = 12$) indicated service provider, and 1.4% ($n = 5$) indicated a parent or parent-in-law.

TABLE 4 Current Caregiving and Care Recipient by Age, Sexual Orientation, and Gender Identity

Variable	Current Caregiver			Care Recipient								
	Yes %	No %	Total n	Partner %	Spouse %	Child %	Parent %	Grandchild %	Other Relative %	Friend/ Neighbor %	Other %	Total n
Total	22.2	77.8	454	16.8	2.0	5.0	40.6	2.0	11.9	30.7	4.0	114
Age	22.2	77.8	454	16.8	2.0	5.0	40.6	2.0	11.9	30.7	4.0	114
48–54	21.5	78.5	130	17.9	0.0	3.6	50.0	0.0	10.7	25.0	3.6	31
55–61	22.6	77.4	208	12.8	2.1	2.1	48.9	2.1	14.9	23.4	4.3	52
65–74	22.1	77.9	95	23.8	4.8	9.5	19.0	4.8	0.0	52.4	4.8	25
75+	23.8	76.2	21	20.0	0.0	20.0	0.0	0.0	40.0	40.0	0.0	6
Sexual orientation	22.3	77.7	452[a]	16.8	2.0	5.0	40.6	2.0	11.9	30.7	4.0	114
Gay man	16.1	83.9	180	24.1	0.0	0.0	41.4	0.0	13.8	31.0	6.9	34
Lesbian	24.4	75.6	217	15.1	1.9	5.7	37.7	1.9	11.3	32.1	3.8	58
Bisexual woman	50.0	50.0	22	9.1	0.0	9.1	54.5	9.1	18.2	18.2	0.0	13
Bisexual man	25.0	75.0	16	0.0	25.0	0.0	75.0	0.0	0.0	25.0	0.0	5
Queer/other	23.5	76.5	17	25.0	0.0	25.0	0.0	0.0	0.0	50.0	0.0	4
Gender identity	22.1	77.9	452[b]	17.0	2.0	4.0	41.0	2.0	12.0	31.0	4.0	113
Transgender woman	36.4	63.6	22	12.5	0.0	12.5	37.5	0.0	12.5	37.5	0.0	9
Transgender man	26.7	73.3	15	25.0	0.0	0.0	50.0	0.0	25.0	25.0	0.0	5
Cisgender woman	25.7	74.3	230	15.3	1.7	5.1	39.0	3.4	11.9	30.5	3.4	65
Cisgender man	15.7	84.3	185	20.7	3.4	0.0	44.8	0.0	10.3	31.0	6.9	34

Note. Participants were allowed to "select all that apply" to indicate all those they care for. The total ($n = 114$) is greater than the number of people who indicated they provide care to another because of this. Eleven people selected two individuals they care for and 1 person selected three. For this table, the number of people in the first column of data is used as the denominator for the percentages in the columns indicating for whom care is provided.

[a] $\chi^2(3, N = 452) = 11.01$, $p < .05$ (for this analysis, those who indicated they were bisexual women or bisexual men were combined into one group: when they were separate, three cells in the chi-square analysis had expected values < 5, which was 30% of the cells; when bisexual women and bisexual men were combined into one group, there was only one cell with an expected value < 5, which was 12.5%). [b] $\chi^2(2, N = 452) = 8.41$, $p < .05$ (for this analysis, those who indicated they were transgender women or transgender men were combined into one group; when they were separate, two cells in the chi-square analysis had expected values < 5, which was 25% of the cells; when transgender women and transgender men were combined into one group, there no cells with an expected value < 5).

TABLE 5 Available Caregiver and Primary Caregiver by Age, Sexual Orientation, and Gender Identity

| | Available Caregiver | | | Who Would Be Your Primary Caregiver? | | | | | | | |
Variable	Yes %	No %	Total n	Partner %	Spouse %	Child %	Parent %	Other/Relative %	Friend/Neighbor %	Service Provider %	Total n
Total	78.3	21.7	456	59.0	11.0	5.6	1.4	5.6	13.8	3.4	354
Age	78.3	21.7	456	59.0	11.0	5.6	1.4	5.6	13.8	3.4	354[a]
48–54	78.5	21.5	130	59.4	10.9	2.0	3.0	7.9	13.9	3.0	101
55–64	77.3	22.7	211	61.1	14.2	3.1	1.2	3.7	14.8	1.9	162
65–74	78.9	21.1	95	60.0	2.7	14.7	0.0	8.0	9.3	5.3	75
75+	85.0	15.0	20	31.3	18.8	12.5	0.0	0.0	25	12.5	16
Sexual orientation	78.2	21.8	454	59.4	10.8	5.4	1.4	5.7	13.9	3.4	352[b]
Gay man	72.9	27.1	181	49.2	6.1	5.3	3.8	9.8	19.7	6.1	132
Lesbian	81.2	18.8	218	71.8	8.6	4.0	0.0	3.4	10.9	1.1	174
Bisexual woman	86.4	13.6	22	57.9	21.1	15.8	0.0	0.0	5.3	0.0	19
Bisexual man	87.5	12.5	16	21.4	50.0	7.1	0.0	7.1	14.3	0.0	14
Queer/other	76.5	23.5	17	38.5	30.8	7.7	0.0	0.0	7.7	15.4	13
Gender Identity	78.4	21.6	454	59.2	10.8	5.7	1.4	5.7	13.9	3.4	353[c]
Transgender woman	82.6	17.4	23	57.9	15.8	10.5	0.0	10.5	5.3	0.0	19
Transgender man	60.0	40.0	15	22.2	33.3	0.0	0.0	11.1	22.2	11.1	9
Cisgender woman	82.2	17.8	230	69.4	10.2	5.4	0.0	2.2	10.8	2.2	186
Cisgender man	74.7	25.3	186	48.2	9.4	5.8	3.6	9.4	18.7	5.0	139

[a] $\chi^2(6, N = 354) = 14.93, p < .05$ (for this analysis, three groups of caregivers were created: partner or spouse, other family, and others; when they were separate, 12 cells in the chi-square analysis had expected values < 5, which was 50% of the cells; when these three groups of caregivers were used, there were 2 cells with an expected value < 5, which was 16.7%). [b] $\chi^2(4, N = 352) = 23.46, p < .01$ (for this analysis, two groups of caregivers were created: partner or spouse and others; when they were separate, 18 cells in the chi-square analysis had expected values < 5, which was 60% of the cells; when these two groups of caregivers were used, there were 2 cells with an expected value < 5, which was 20%). [c] $\chi^2(3, N = 353) = 19.37, p < .01$ (for this analysis, two groups of caregivers were created: partner or spouse and others; when they were separate, 13 cells in the chi-square analysis had expected values < 5, which was 54.2% of the cells; when these two groups of caregivers were used, there was 1 cell with an expected value < 5, which was 12.5%).

When looking at age, three groups of available care providers were created: partner or spouse, other family (i.e., parent, child, or other relative), and others. The pattern of responses for care providers was related to age, $\chi^2(6, N = 354) = 14.93, p < .05$.

When conducting chi-square analyses with sexual orientation and gender identity, the categories used for caregiver were partner or spouse and other. This further collapsing into two categories was done to reach the criterion that no more than 20% of cells in the chi-square analyses have < 5 expected values. The pattern of response to who would serve as caregiver was significantly related to sexual orientation, $\chi^2(4, N = 352) = 23.46$, $p < .01$; and gender identity, $\chi^2(3, N = 353) = 19.37, p < .01$.

Significantly more gay men, than what was expected by chance, indicated their primary caregiver would be someone other than a partner or spouse (44.7%; $n = 59$; SRS $= 3.1$), whereas significantly fewer gay men indicated their primary care giver would be a partner or spouse (55.3%; $n = 73$; SRS $= -2.0$). Significantly fewer lesbians indicated that someone other than a partner or spouse would serve as their caregiver (19.5%; $n = 34$; SRS $= -2.5$).

Significantly fewer cisgender women indicated that they considered someone other than a partner or spouse to be their primary care giver (20.4%; $n = 38$; SRS $= -2.4$), whereas significantly more cisgender men indicated their primary care giver would be someone other than a partner or spouse (42.4%; $n = 59$; SRS $= 2.7$).

Enough close friends and caregiving. The pattern of responses about having a care provider for oneself is related to having enough close friends, $\chi^2(1, N = 453) = 7.49, p < .01$. Significantly more people than expected who indicated they do not feel they have enough close friends also indicated they do not have someone who would take care of them if they were sick or unable to care for themselves (29.1%; $n = 46$; SRS $= 2.0$). Similarly, 82% ($n = 242$) of people who indicated they feel they do have enough close friends also indicated they have someone who would take care of them.

DISCUSSION

As an individual ages, having an informal caregiver is a key predictor for remaining in the community and this need is most often met by a spouse, adult daughter or daughter-in-law. This circumstance points to the unique characteristics of LGBT caregiving that are highlighted in the results of this study: LGBT individuals are less likely to be married or partnered and less likely to have children than the general population. A comparison of the study results with those of the general population 50 years and older using the most recent Survey of Older Minnesotans for the Twin Cities Metro Area (Minnesota Board on Aging, 2005), suggest (a) diminished access to traditional sources of caregivers and (b) nontraditional caregiving patterns that reflect the importance of the chosen family for successful LGBT aging.

Access to Caregivers

While a spouse and adult children are primary sources of informal caregiver support, many LGBT midlife and older adults may not have these relationships. LGBT older adults were less likely to have a partner or spouse (59.5%) compared to the Twin Cities population (65.6%) and almost $2\frac{1}{2}$ times less likely to have children (35.4% compared to 84.5%; Minnesota Board on Aging, 2005).

A more nuanced look at these results shows gay men and cisgender men were more likely to be single, and lesbians and cisgendered women were less likely to be single. It is interesting to note that lesbians, bisexual women, bisexual men, transgender women, and cisgender women reported being partnered at rates higher than the general population.

Similarly, gay men were less likely to have children while those over 65 years of age, bisexual men and bisexual women and transwomen were more likely to have children. This type of closer look at who within the LGBT community is more or less likely to have access to traditional caregiving support points to the diversity of experience and resources and how "one size will not fit all" when planning for successful LGBT aging.

It is interesting to note that the overall rate of having a partner or spouse was considerably higher than the 44.3% reported by the recent *Aging and Health Report* (Fredriksen-Goldsen et al., 2011). However, looking at the baby boomer cohort of this sample (48–64 years of age), 59.7% reported having a partner or spouse, a rate that is consistent with the 58% partnered rate found in the MetLife (2010) LGBT baby boomer study. Whether these represent regional or some other source of variation is an interesting empirical question and remains to be seen.

Caregiving Patterns

Available caregiver. LGBT older adults were less likely to have an available caregiver (75.5%) than the general population (89.5%). Although there were no significant differences in availability of a caregiver by age, sexual orientation and gender identity, gay men, cisgender men, and transgender men reported the lowest rates of available caregivers, whereas bisexual women and bisexual men reported rates approaching those of the larger population. Because having a caregiver is a key indicator for remaining in your home and community (Miller & Weissert, 2000; Spillman & Long, 2009), those populations within the LGBT community with lower available caregiver rates may be at greater risk for long-term residential placements.

Of those respondents who were able to identify a potential caregiver, 73.1% (252) identified a partner (not a spouse), friend, or neighbor—that is, they identified someone not legally related to them. Non-related caregivers have fewer caregiver support resources available to them through the caregiver support network and therefore may experience greater stress than legally related caregivers. High caregiver stress is tied to poorer outcomes for the caregiver (e.g., financial and retirement security, emotional and physical health) and is a predictor for nursing home placement for the care receiver (Spillman & Long, 2009).

Hierarchy of seeking assistance. The pattern of seeking caregiving assistance found in the larger community typically follows a hierarchy starting with a spouse, then child, other relatives and finally approaching friends and neighbors (Shanas, 1980), but may not be as applicable in the non-heteronormative LGBT community (Barker, 2006). As observed in the larger community, almost all (96.4%) individuals reporting a partner or spouse also identified their partner or spouse as an available primary caregiver. However, LGBT individuals without a partner most frequently identified friends and neighbors (46.2%), followed by children (19.7%), other relatives (18.7%), service providers (9.9%) and parents (5.5%). Because approximately two in five members of the LGBT population are without a partner or spouse, caregiving by friends and neighbors becomes a significant segment of the caregiving resource.

Current caregiving. LGBT older adults were serving as caregivers almost twice as often as the general population (22.3% compared to 12.5%) and caring for friends and neighbors more than twice as frequently (30.7% compared to 13.2%; Minnesota Board on Aging, 2005). These overall rates of LGBT caregiving and specific caregiving for friends and neighbors are similar to the findings of the Health and Aging Report (Fredriksen-Goldsen et al., 2011), which found 27% of the older LGBT population serving as caregivers and of these caregivers, 32% were caring for friends and neighbors. In the baby boomer cohort of this sample, 22.1% were serving as caregivers of which 24.0% provided care to friends and neighbors. This is consistent with the MetLife (2010) findings, which were 21% and 22%, respectively.

The caregiving and potential caregiver patterns observed in this study point to the importance of friends and neighbors in successful LGBT aging. Three-fourths indicated they had a chosen family defined as a group of people to whom you are emotionally close and consider "family," although you are not biologically or legally related. Friends and neighbors close enough to be identified as potential primary caregivers might also be within one's chosen family. Further, those who reported not having enough close friends were more likely to report not having an available caregiver.

Family acceptance. It is important to note 63.7% (284) of LGBT older adults reported their families of origin to be extremely accepting or very accepting of their life as an LGBT person. Presumably, these individuals might seek and find within their family of origin a caregiver for themselves or support for their role as caregivers to others. However, the 10.1% who reported their families of origin to be not very accepting or not at all accepting will most likely need to find support from other sources (e.g., chosen family members or professional services). In the MetLife (2010) baby boomer study, 14% reported families that were not at all accepting or not very accepting, and one-half reported families to be very accepting or extremely accepting. The current study found baby boomer family acceptance rates somewhat more promising at 9.2% and 61.8%, respectively.

Women and caregiving. The caregiver patterns observed in this sample point to an important similarity to the general population: Women were more likely to serve as caregivers. Two-thirds of the caregivers in this study were women, and one-half of bisexual women were providing care. Both cisgender men and gay men reported the lowest rate of caregiving. The higher rate of female caregiving agrees with the findings of the *Aging and Heath Report* (Fredriksen-Goldsen et al., 2011), but is in contrast to the MetLife (2010) baby boomer study which found men were as likely as women to be caregivers.

Risk indicators. LGBT older adults were more likely to live alone (39.5%) compared to the general population (24.5%; Minnesota Board on Aging, 2005). Living alone and lack of a caregiver are recognized as critical indicators for risk of nursing home placement and are two of the seven risk factors used in the Live Well at Home Rapid Screening Project developed by the Minnesota Department of Human Services and deployed across the state (Gaugler, Boldischar, Vujovich, & Yahnke, 2011; Gaugler, Krichbaum, & Wyman, 2009). The presence of two or more of the seven risk factors identifies an individual at higher risk for institutionalization. As a result, intensive options counseling occurs to mitigate the risk through diversion support services. In this study, 82 individuals (18%) reported they both lived alone and did not have an available caregiver.

Policy Implications

The vital role of informal caregiving in the lives of older adults has been recognized by the federal government, most notably with the 2000 enactment of the Older Americans Act National Family Caregiver Support Program (NFCSP). Caregivers offer a wide variety of services to support older adults including assistance with personal cares and activities of daily living, grocery shopping, and home and yard care. This care is recognized as saving billions of dollars to the public sector annually. Programs such as NFCSP provide funding to support caregivers providing services to older adults through education, coaching and ancillary services. However, recent research has shown that home and community based service providers lack education about the unique needs of LGBT older adults in general, let alone LGBT caregiving specifically (Knochel et al., 2012; Moone & Cagle, 2011).

A further complication in accessing caregiver support services is often the very definition of "caregiver" adopted by policymakers and service providers. LGBT older adults were more likely to identify a non-relation (i.e., partner or friend) to serve as a caregiver than a legal relation. Fortunately, the definition of caregiver within the NFCSP recognizes the complex and diverse nature of caregiver relationships and includes non-related caregivers. All individuals in a primary caregiving relationship can benefit from the caregiver support programs throughout the United States funded by the NFCSP. This covers the (at least) 10% of caregivers not legally related to the person receiving care and includes LGBT caregivers. However, the practice of recognizing and respecting non-related caregiving relationships is not universally accepted. In a report from the National Senior Citizens Law Center (2011) entitled *Stories from the Field*, it was found that 11% of LGBT residents of nursing homes had staff refuse to accept a power of attorney, often one of the most important documents in LGBT older adults' lives. The same percentage of residents had experienced a restriction of visitors.

In this study, almost 17% of caregivers reported caring for a partner. State policies vary in their recognition of same-sex relationships and most often policies available to legally married couples are not available to non-married same-sex couples. A most recent example is the clarification by the federal Department of Health and Human Services regarding the Medicaid spousal impoverishment provision. This provision allows one spouse to receive Medicaid funding while residing in a nursing home and protects the community-dwelling spouse from impoverishment through Medicaid spend downs and liens. In this instance, the federal government acknowledged impoverishment protections of same-sex relationships only in instances where states recognized the relationship (National Senior Citizens Law Center, 2011). This is an example of how narrow definitions of caregiving relationships and the failure to recognize non-heteronormative family structures limit caregiver supports available to LGBT older adults.

Although the federal government has made significant strides in raising awareness of the unique needs of LGBT older adults through the National Research Center on LGBT Aging, there is still substantial work that needs to occur with regard to LGBT caregiving. In addition, research is needed to further examine (a) the role of families of choice in the care of LGBT older adults and (b) caregiver support providers' knowledge and understanding of LGBT chosen family support systems. Further advocacy and education is needed with mainstream service providers specifically regarding the complex nature of caregiving in the LGBT community.

Strengths and Limitations

This community survey drew a large number of responses and closely approximated the ethnic and racial distribution of the Twin Cities Metropolitan Area. However, the predominance of White non-Latinos in the region's 48 and older age demographic (93.2%) makes it difficult to draw conclusions about communities of color. Similarly, the experiences of smaller segments within the LGBT population (e.g., bisexual, gender-nonconforming individuals) are not well understood through this sample.

Recruitment for the survey was primarily accomplished online through LGBT community organizations who directed their constituents to the survey link. By distributing the survey in this manner, the resulting convenience sample may have over represented community members who are more comfortable with their LGBT identity (i.e., out enough to belong to 1 or more LGBT groups), socially connected and less isolated, and computer literate or those with greater Internet access than the larger population.

Further, the survey did not specify "legal" when referring to spouse or marriage in several questions. One respondent, when asked to provide a multiple choice answer that included selecting between a spouse or a partner, wrote, "I'm confused, my partner is my spouse. I'm not sure what you want." Due to the dynamic state of same-sex marriage across the United States, references to marriage within the LGBT community require greater specificity.

CONCLUSION

This study contributes to the overall understanding of LGBT aging and helps researchers, policymakers and service providers respond to the needs of this poorly documented and poorly understood community. It also highlights the high rate of caregiving, as well as the high rate of nontraditional caregiving patterns within the LGBT community and suggests opportunities to create support services that truly support LGBT caregivers. Service providers need to fully understand the extent to which the NFCSP can be used to assist LGBT clients. They also need to create welcoming supportive services and make those services known to the LGBT community. Policymakers wishing to create mechanisms that sustain the largest number of individuals in the community and prevent nursing home placements, should consider ways to more fully support the 10% of caregivers that are non-kin, perhaps through expansion of caregiver supports that are currently limited to legal kin including the Family Medical Leave Act, equivalent Medicaid spend-downs, Social Security benefits, bereavement leave, and automatic inheritance of jointly owned real estate and personal property (Fredriksen-Goldsen & Hoy-Ellis, 2007).

Until recently, with the exception of the MetLife (2010) *Still Out, Still Aging* study and the *Aging and Health Report* (Fredriksen-Goldsen et al., 2011), almost all data about LGBT aging has been gathered in local LGBT aging needs assessments such as the survey that provided the sample for this study. The appearance of national data sets might suggest that local needs assessments have run their course. However, until questions about sexual orientation and gender identity become regular demographic components of national surveys, including the U.S. Census, local surveys will continue to play an important role in developing an understanding of LGBT aging.

FUNDING

This study was funded, in part, by Greater Twin Cities United Way and PFund Foundation.

NOTE

1. Cisgender describes individuals who have a match between the gender they were assigned at birth, their bodies, and their personal identity; and is the compliment of transgender (see Schilt & Westbrook, 2009).

REFERENCES

AARP Public Policy Institute. (2011). *Valuing the invaluable: Growing contributions and costs of family caregiving.* Washington, DC: Author.

Adelman, M., Gurevich, L., de Vries, B., & Blando, J. (2006). Openhouse: Community building and research in the LGBT aging population. In D. Kimmel, T. Rose, & S. David (Eds.), *Lesbian, gay, bisexual, and transgender aging: Research and clinical perspectives* (pp. 247–264). New York, NY: Columbia University Press.

Barker, J. C. (2002). Neighbors, friends, and other nonkin caregivers of community-living dependent elders. *Journals of Gerontology Series B: Psychological Sciences & Social Sciences,* 57B(3), 158.

Barker, J. C., Herdt, G., & de Vries, B. (2006). Social supports in the lives of lesbians and gay men at midlife and later. *Sexuality Research & Social policy: Journal of the NSRC,* 3(2), 1–23.

Beeler, J., Rawls, T., Herdt, G., & Cohler, B. (1999). The needs of older lesbians and gay men in Chicago. *Journal of Gay and Lesbian Social Services,* 9(1), 31–49.

Bell, S. A., Bern-Klug, M., Kramer, K. W. O., & Saunders, J. B. (2010). Most nursing home social service directors lack training in working with lesbian, gay and bisexual residents. *Social Work in Health Care,* 49, 814–831.

Brotman, S., Ryan, B., Collins, S., Chamberland, L., Cormier, R., Julien, D., & . . .Richard, B. (2007). Coming out to care: Caregivers of gay and lesbian seniors in Canada. *Gerontologist,* 47, 490–503.

Brotman, S., Ryan, B., & Cormier, R. (2003). The health and social service needs of gay and lesbian elders and their families in Canada. *Gerontologist,* 43, 192–201.

Cantor, M. H., Brennan, M., & Shippy, R. A. (2004). *Caregiving among older lesbian, gay, bisexual and transgender New Yorkers.* New York, NY: Policy Institute of the National Gay and Lesbian Task Force.

Clark, M. E., Landers, S., Linde, R., & Sperber, J. (2001). The GLBT health access project: A state-funded effort to improve access to care. *American Journal of Public Health,* 91, 895–896.

Croghan, C., Mertens, A., Yoakam, J., & Edwards, N. (2003, April). *GLBT senior needs assessment*. Poster presented at the Aging in America conference, Chicago, IL.

Croghan, C., Moone, R., & Olson, A. (2012). *Twin Cities LGBT aging needs assessment survey*. Minneapolis, MN: Greater Twin Cities United Way and PFund Foundation.

de Vries, B. (2006). Home at the end of the rainbow. *Generations, 29*(4), 64–69.

de Vries, B. (2011). LGBT aging: Research and policy directions. *Public Policy and Aging Report, 21*(3), 34–35.

de Vries, B., & Hoctel, P. (2006). The family–friends of older gay men and lesbians. In N. Teunis & G. Herdt (Eds.), *Sexual inequalities and social justice* (pp. 213–232). Berkeley, CA: University of California Press.

Fredriksen, K. I. (1999). Family caregiving responsibilities among lesbians and gay men. *Social Work, 44*, 142–155.

Fredriksen-Goldsen, K. I., & Hoy-Ellis, C. P. (2007). Caregiving with pride: An introduction. *Journal of Gay & Lesbian Social Services*, 18(3/4), 1–13.

Fredriksen-Goldsen, K. I., Kim, H.-J., Emlet, C. A., Muraco, A., Erosheva, E. A., Hoy-Ellis, C. P., . . .Petry, H. (2011). *Aging and health report: Disparities and resilience among lesbian, gay, bisexual, and transgender older adults*. Seattle, WA: Institute for Multigenerational Health.

Gaugler, J., Boldischar, M., Vujovich, J., & Yahnke, P. (2011). The Minnesota Live Well at Home Project: Screening and client satisfaction. *Home Health Care Service Quarterly, 30*(2), 63–83.

Gaugler, J., Krichbaum, K., & Wyman, J. (2009). Predictors of nursing home admission for persons with dementia. *Medical Care, 47*, 191–198.

Grant, J. M., Mottet, L. A., & Tanis, J. (2010). *Injustice at every turn: A report of the national transgender discrimination survey*. Washington, DC: National Center for Transgender Equality and National Gay and Lesbian Task Force. Retrieved from http://www.thetaskforce.org/downloads/reports/reports/ntds_full.pdf

Grossman, A. H., d'Augelli, A. R., & Hershberger, S. L. (2000). Social support networks of lesbian, gay and bisexual adults 60 years of age and older. *Journals of Gerontology Series B: Psychological Sciences and Social Sciences, 55B*(3), 171–179.

Hillier, S., & Barrow, G. (2010). *Aging, individual and society* (9th ed.). Belmont, CA: Wadsworth.

Hughes, M. (2009). Lesbian and gay people's concerns about ageing and accessing services. *Australian Social Work, 62*, 186–201.

Institute of Medicine. (2011). *The health of lesbian, gay, bisexual and transgender people: Building a foundation for better understanding*. Washington, DC: National Academies Press.

Jackson, N. C., Johnson, M. J., & Roberts, R. (2008). The potential impact of discrimination fears of older gays, lesbians, bisexuals and transgender individuals living in small to moderate sized cities on long-term health care. *Journal of Homosexuality, 54*(3), 325–339.

Knochel, K. A., Croghan, C. F., Moone, R., & Quam, J. (2012). Training, geography and provision of aging services to lesbian, gay, bisexual, and transgender older adults. *Journal of Gerontological Social Work, 55*, 426–443.

Knochel, K. A., Quam, J. K., & Croghan, C. F. (2011). Are old lesbian and gay people well served? Understanding the perceptions, preparation, and experiences of aging service providers. *Journal of Applied Gerontology, 30,* 370–389.

Logie, C., Bridge, T. J., & Bridge, P. D. (2008). Evaluating the phobias, attitudes, and cultural competence of Master of Social Work students toward the LGBT populations. *Journal of Homosexuality, 53*(4), 201–221.

MetLife. (2010). *Still out, still aging: The MetLife study of lesbian, gay, bisexual and transgender baby boomers.* Westport, CT: MetLife Mature Market Institute.

Miller, A. M., & Weissert, W. G. (2000). Predicting elderly people's risk for nursing home placement, hospitalization, functional impairment and mortality: A synthesis. *Medical Care Research Review, 57,* 259–297.

Minnesota Board on Aging. (2005). *Survey of older Minnesotans.* St. Paul, MN: Minnesota Board on Aging. Retrieved from http://www.mnaging.org/advisor/survey/SOM2005Tables.pdf

Moone, R., & Cagle, J. G. (2011). A content analysis of Aging Network conference proceedings. *Educational Gerontology, 37,* 955–1008.

National Alliance for Caregiving and AARP. (2009). *Caregiving in the U.S. 2009.* Bethesda, MD: Author.

National Gay and Lesbian Task Force. (2012). *Relationship recognition for same-sex couples in the U.S.* Washington, DC: National Gay and Lesbian Task Force. Retrieved from http://www.thetaskforce.org/downloads/reports/issue_maps/rel_recog_6_28_11_color.pdf

National Senior Citizens Law Center, National Gay and Lesbian Task Force, SAGE, Lamda Legal, National Center for Lesbian Rights, and National Center for Transgender Equality. (2011). *Stories from the field: LGBT older adults in long-term care facilities.* Washington, DC: Author.

Schilt, K., & Westbrook, L. (2009). Doing gender, doing heteronormativity: "Gender normals," transgender people, and the social maintenance of heterosexuality. *Gender & Society, 23,* 440–464.

Services and Advocacy for GLBT Elders. (2011). *Spousal impoverishment protections initiative.* New York, NY: Author.

Shanas, E. (1980). Older people and their families: The new pioneers. *Journal of Marriage & the Family, 42,* 9.

Spillman, B., & Long S. (2009). Does high caregiver stress predict nursing home entry? *Inquiry, 46,* 140–161.

Steele, L. S., Tinmouth, J. M., & Lu, A. (2006). Regular health care use by lesbians: A path analysis of predictive factors. *Family Practice, 23,* 631–636.

U.S. Census Bureau. (2012). *American fact finder. Minneapolis–St. Paul–Bloomington, MN–WI Metro Area, Metropolitan Statistical Area.* Washington, DC: U.S. Census Bureau. Retrieved from http://www.factfinder2.census.gov

Willging, C. E., Salvador, M., & Kano, M. (2006). Unequal treatment: Mental health care for sexual and gender minority groups in a rural state. *Psychiatric Services, 57,* 867–870.

Witten, T. M. (2009). Graceful exits: Intersection of aging, transgender identities, and the family/community. *Journal of GLBT Family Studies, 5*(1/2), 35–61.

The Greater St. Louis LGBT Health and Human Services Needs Assessment: An Examination of the Silent and Baby Boom Generations

MEGHAN JENKINS MORALES, MSW, M. DENISE KING, PhD,
HATTIE HILER, BA, MARTIN S. COOPWOOD, MS,
and SHERRILL WAYLAND, MSW
SAGE Metro St. Louis, St. Louis, Missouri, USA

This study sought to understand differences and similarities between lesbian, gay, bisexual, and transgender (LGBT) Baby Boomers and members of the Silent generation in the greater St. Louis region in relation to perceived barriers to service use, LGBT identity disclosure, experiences of violence and victimization, and mental health. An online survey was completed by 118 Baby Boomers and 33 Silents. Baby Boomers were found to perceive more barriers to health care and legal services, have fewer legal documents in place, feel less safe in their communities, and have experienced an increased rate of verbal harassment compared to their predecessors. Differences may be attributed to higher levels of LGBT identity disclosure among Baby Boomers across their lifetime. These findings support the current work of Services and Advocacy for GLBT Elders Metro St. Louis, with implications for other communities, and shed light on the need for continued advancement in the development and implementation of programs as LGBT Baby Boomers age.

Lesbian, gay, bisexual, and transgender (LGBT) older adults are described as an "invisible" or "hidden" segment of the aging population (Blando, 2001; Brotman, Ryan, & Cormier, 2003; Butler, 2004; D'Augelli, Grossman,

Hershberger, & O'Connell, 2001; Hash & Cramer, 2003; Shankle, Maxwell, Katzman, & Landers, 2003). Brotman et al. characterized this invisibility as a defense mechanism used to combat further discrimination due to age and sexual orientation. Considering the broader context, Cahill (2002) noted that a consequence of this invisibility is disregard for the needs of LGBT older adults.

Research estimates that 3% to 8% of the general population identifies as LGBT (Institute of Medicine, 2011). According to the U.S. Census Bureau (2010), the greater St. Louis region is home to 955,989 adults over the age of 50. Based on these estimates, it is projected that between 28,680 and 76,479 LGBT adults aged 50 and older live in the greater St. Louis region. The journey to unveil the needs of the St. Louis LGBT older adult population began in 2008 with the formation of SAGE (Services and Advocacy for GLBT Elders) Metro St. Louis.

SAGE Metro St. Louis is a local affiliate of the national SAGE network. SAGE works to enhance the quality of life of LGBT older adults through service, advocacy, and community awareness. In addition to the experiences of local task force members, research which informed the early services and programs largely came from two reports: *Outing Age* (Cahill, South, & Spade, 2000) conducted by the National Gay and Lesbian Task Force and *Out and Aging* (MetLife, 2006). SAGE used the reports early on to estimate needed services and assist in the strategic planning process which led to program implementation. Although the reports were helpful, information was needed at the local level to ensure the needs of LGBT older adults in the SAGE service area were understood.

Also established in 2008, One St. Louis is a non-profit volunteer service organization that works to fill the gaps in services for the LGBT and other under-served communities in the St. Louis area. In 2010, SAGE partnered with One St. Louis to implement a local needs assessment. This research team developed the St. Louis needs assessment modeled after the 2009 LGBT Health and Human Services Needs Assessment conducted in New York State (Frazer, 2009).

This study is based on findings from the 2010 Greater St. Louis Health and Human Services Needs Assessment of LGBT adults over the age of 50. Information was gathered on perceived and actual barriers to service use, mental health status, experiences of violence and victimization, and LGBT identity disclosure. Limited research has examined the heterogeneity of the LGBT older adult population by exploring possible variation between generations. This study also examines potential differences between two cohorts of older LGBT adults; the Baby Boom generation (50–64 years old in 2010) and the Silent generation (65–79 years old in 2010).

The term "Silent Generation" was first coined in a 1951 *Time Magazine* cover story describing the generation born during the Great Depression ("The Younger Generation," 1951). It is generally accepted that the Silent generation came before the Baby Boom generation (Centers for Disease Control, 2009), although researchers differ in their definitions of the age range of the Silent generation (hereafter referred to as the *Silents*). For the purposes of this study, respondents born from 1925 through 1945 are considered members of the Silent generation (Egri & Ralston, 2004). Baby Boomers are defined as persons born from 1946 through 1964 (U.S. Census Bureau, 2011).

BACKGROUND AND LITERATURE REVIEW

Historical context has shaped the lives of LGBT older adults. As noted by Kimmel, Rose, Orel, and Greene (2006) the intersection of social change and historical cohort within the LGBT population is profound. LGBT Silents came of age in a time prior to identity and disclosure as it is known today. The American Psychiatric Association classified homosexuality as a mental disorder until 1973, when the oldest Silents were 42 years old (American Psychiatric Association, 1973). Baby Boomers came of age during major cultural shifts and were the first cohort to experience the LGBT visibility that came with the gay rights movement. During the New York City Stonewall Riots of 1969, the youngest of the Baby Boomer cohort were only five years old.

Unlike the Baby Boomers who followed them, the Silents lacked the critical mass to dominate American society or the workforce. The Silent generation grew up during a time when adherence to the ethics and morals of the dominate culture defined the character of an individual, authority was respected, and conformity was seen as the key to success (G. Williams, 2002). Although they were born during the Great Depression, the Silent generation experienced a booming post World War II economy and many could rely on fixed-benefit pension plans during retirement (Salkowitz, 2008). Members of the Baby Boom generation are working longer compared to the Silent generation and pathways out of the workforce have become more complex over time (Johnson, Butrica, & Mommaerts, 2010). The number one concern of LGBT Baby Boomers as they age is financial stability (MetLife, 2010), with lesbians reporting greater financial concerns than gay men (MetLife, 2010; Orel, 2004).

In 2011, the first Baby Boomers turned 65 years old. It has been projected that Baby Boomers are more likely to view retirement positively, be proactive about the aging processes, and challenge restrictions through legislative action and political organization (Hooyman & Kiyak, 2011). These differences will change the way future cohorts experience aging, just as the experience of this generation has affected so many societal institutions (Dychtwald, 2000). It is helpful from theoretical, practice, and policy dimensions to understand the needs and perspectives of the current cohort of older adults and anticipate upcoming changes with the appearance of the Baby Boom generation.

However, the majority of previous research has not specifically examined cohort or generational differences within the LGBT older adult community. The findings from prior research on the general LGBT adult population provide a helpful foundation when working to understand potential differences between generations. Previous research examining violence and victimization, mental health and barriers to services help explain the unique challenges that LGBT Baby Boomers and members of the Silent generation confront as they age.

Violence & Victimization

LGBT individuals have been found to be at greater risk for violence and victimization over the life course than heterosexual counterparts (Balsam, Rothblum, & Beauchaine, 2005; Corliss, Cochran, & Mays, 2002; Fredriksen-Goldsen et al., 2011). Victimization based on actual or perceived sexual orientation or gender identity is often a result of visibility due to nonconforming gender expression or LGBT identity disclosure (D'Augelli, Hershberger, & Pilkington, 1998). An association between earlier self-disclosure of sexual orientation and more experiences of victimization has also been found (D'Augelli et al., 2001).

Grossman, D' Augelli, and O'Connell (2001), using a national sample of 416 lesbian, gay, or bisexual (LGB) adults over the age of 60, found that 63% experienced verbal abuse, 29% received threats of physical violence, and 29% reported being victimized by someone who threatened to disclose their sexual orientation. In a sample of 402 transgender adults, Lombardi, Wilchins, Priesing, and Malouf (2002) found that over one-half of the respondents experienced some form of harassment or violence over their lifetime, with one-fourth of them experiencing a violent incident. Findings from the *Aging and Health Report,* a national project with 2,560 LGBT older adult respondents, indicated that two-thirds had experienced verbal harassment and 43% reported physical violence (Fredriksen-Goldsen et al., 2011).

Mental Health

A significant relation has been reported between victimization status and previous suicide attempts among LGB older adults (D'Augelli et al., 2001). Researchers have also found that experiences of discrimination and expectations of discrimination contribute to loneliness among LGB older adults (Grossman et al., 2001; Kuyper & Fokkema, 2010). Evidence also suggests that LGBT individuals suffer from more mental distress compared to their heterosexual counterparts (Cochran & Mays, 2000; Gilman et al., 2001; Meyer,

2003; Sandfort, De Graaf, Bijl, & Schnabel, 2001). Researchers have attributed these elevated rates of mental distress to the effects of prejudice, stigma, and discrimination, which create a stressful environment for LGBT individuals (Friedman, 1999; Grant, 2010; Meyer, 2003). Negative mental health outcomes within the LGBT older adult community can be attributed to the accumulated effect of enduring a lifetime of stigma (Institute of Medicine, 2011), which can assume multiple forms.

Meyer (2003) elaborated on the conceptual framework of *minority stress* to explain the higher prevalence of mental disorders within the LGBT community. Minority stress is described as chronic stress related to stigmatization and actual experiences of discrimination and violence that can lead to adverse mental health outcomes for LGBT individuals (Meyer, 2003). Given the heterogeneity within the LGBT population, the impact of minority stress on an individual with multiple minority identities will differ from the effect of minority stress on a gay White male. Previous studies support the role of minority stress in relation to the mental health outcomes of LGB older adults; however, little evidence specific to the transgender community exists (D'Augelli et al., 2001; Grossman et al., 2001; Kuyper & Fokkema, 2010).

Barriers to Services

LGBT older adults are also less likely to seek supportive services which may in turn leave them at risk for social isolation and depression (Butler, 2004; Cahill, 2000). In a 2006 study, less than one-half of gay and lesbian Baby Boomers were confident that health care professionals would treat them with dignity and respect (MetLife, 2006). Institutionalized homophobia and heteronormativity create potential discriminatory action and practices that further isolate and promote fearful reactions of LGBT older adults (Butler 2004; Cahill et al., 2000; Shankle et al., 2003).

Orel (2004) found that LGB older adults who share their sexual orientation with their primary health care provider report more positive experiences, but due to fear of discrimination, many LGB older adults are hesitant to reveal their sexual orientation (King & Dabelko-Schoeny, 2009). When confronted with homophobic and heteronormative institutions, some LGBT older adults may "return to the closet" as a defense mechanism (Cahill, 2002; Phillips & Marks, 2006).

Having greater access to service systems may reduce the adverse mental health outcomes that can accompany perceived and actual experiences of discrimination for LGBT older adults. Accomplishing this task would require a change in attitudes, increased training, and adoption of inclusive practices and policies (Anetzberger, Ishler, Mostade, & Blair, 2004; Brotman et al., 2003; Butler, 2004; Cahill, 2002; Cahill et al., 2000; Maccio & Doueck, 2002; Reingold & Burros, 2004; Shankle et al., 2003; Steinsvåg, Sandkjaer, & Størksen, 2004; Ward, Vass, Aggarwal, Garfield, & Cybyk, 2005).

Identification of barriers to services at the local level can help target programs and advocacy efforts to meet the specific needs of LGBT older adults.

METHOD

The needs assessment was conducted in collaboration between SAGE and One Saint Louis, which were both established in 2008. As new nonprofits, it was essential to gather baseline data on the needs of the LGBT community and older LGBT adults in particular. The purpose of the assessment was to understand the health and human services needs of LGBT individuals in the St. Louis area to identify and support the implementation of programs and services specific to the identified needs. The needs assessment received internal review board approval through Washington University Human Research Protection Office. The survey instrument used for this needs assessment was developed by the research team and modeled after the first statewide LGBT needs assessment in New York conducted by the Empire State Pride Agenda Foundation and the New York State LGBT Health and Human Services Network (Frazer, 2009).

Procedure

The online program Survey Monkey was used to distribute the survey and collect data over the course of 6 months, from June to November, 2010. The survey was open to adults over the age of 18. A brief introduction explained the purpose of the survey and potential risks that were involved. The statement, "Completing this survey indicates your consent," was included in the introduction before respondents began the survey. Convenience sampling and snowballing techniques were used to obtain participants in the target population. Announcements regarding the survey and a link to the survey were distributed through local LGBT organization Web sites, newsletters, listservs, and social media outlets. The survey was sent to over 700 community members through the e-mail lists of SAGE Metro St. Louis and One St. Louis. In addition, the LGBT nonprofit coalition consisting of over 20 nonprofits and social groups in Missouri was asked to assist with the survey distribution.

The purpose of this study was to examine differences and similarities between Baby Boomers and the Silent generation in relation to barriers to service use, LGBT identity disclosure, experiences of violence and victimization, and mental health. Statistical analyses were performed using Statistical Package for the Social Sciences Version 19.0 (SPSS, Inc., Chicago, IL). Bivariate analyses were used to compare Baby Boomers and the Silent generation on several measures. For continuous variables t tests for independent samples and Pearson's correlation coefficient (r) were used and categorical variables were compared using chi-square analyses (chi-square). Gender comparisons were also made using bivariate analyses. When statistical tests were significant, the test statistic and significance are reported. Comparisons of particular interest or those approaching significance are also noted.

Measures

Barriers to services. Barriers to health care and legal services were addressed using Likert-type scales. Respondents were asked to report if a barrier was "no problem at all," "a very slight problem," "somewhat of a problem," or "a major problem." Some of the barriers to health care that were addressed include lack of LGBT friendly support groups, inadequately trained health care and mental health professionals to provide services to LGBT people, and personal financial resources. Barriers to legal services that were addressed include limited knowledge of legal services, access to LGBT friendly attorneys, and personal financial resources. Responses to Likert questions related to service barriers were summed to create a continuous measure as an overall appraisal of perceived barriers to service use.

Questions related to health care insurance, health care service provider and legal documents were also included in the survey instrument. Respondents were asked, "What type of health care insurance do you use to pay for your doctor and hospital bills?" Nine response options were available, ranging from "through my employer," "Medicare or Medicaid," or "none; I don't have health insurance." Another question related to health care service provider type asked, "If you need health care, where do you usually get it?" Again, nine response options were available ranging from "private doctor," to "clinic at a hospital," to "nowhere." Respondents were also asked to respond to the statement, "I have the following legal documents." The instruction was to "check all that apply," with response options including "will," "living will," "power of attorney for finances," "power of attorney for health care," "trust," "none," or "other." For analysis purposes response options were dummy coded to identify individual legal documents that respondents had in place.

LGBT identity disclosure. To assess LGBT identity disclosure, respondents were asked, "How much do you agree or disagree with each of the following statements about being out as a lesbian, gay, bisexual and/or transgender person?" The statements referenced disclosure in relation to family, friends, work, and health care provider; for example, "I am out to my family." A 5-point Likert scale was used, with responses ranging from 4 (*strongly agree*) to 0 (*strongly disagree*). Responses were summed to create an overall measure of LGBT identity disclosure with higher scores indicating greater disclosure.

One question addressed LGBT community involvement: "Last year, how many times did you go to events at an LGBT center or other place that was specifically for LGBT people?" A 5-point Likert-type scale ranging from 0 (*never*) to 4 (*more often than once per month*) was used. Another question asked respondents, "If there was a list of health and human service providers who were certified as being trained in, knowledgeable about, and sensitive to LGBT issues, how likely is it that you would use this list to choose a provider?" Response options included "not at all," "a little bit," "a lot," or "I would only choose those providers who were on this list and met these conditions."

Violence and victimization. Violence and victimization were assessed based on "yes" or "no" responses. Respondents were asked, "Have you ever experienced any of the following that you have reason to believe was motivated by homophobia (fear or dislike of lesbians, gay men or bisexual people) or transphobia (fear or dislike of transgender people)?" The following options were provided for response: "verbal harassment," "neglect by a caregiver," "taken advantage of financially or blackmailed," "property damage or arson," "physical assault," "sexual assault," and "physical assault serious enough to require medical attention." For each type of victimization, respondents had the option to endorse if the incident was due to homophobia, transphobia, or both. In the same "yes" or "no" format, respondents were asked if the incident was reported to the police. Incidents motivated by transphobia were not included in the final analysis due to the small number of endorsements to this item; however, incidents endorsed by transgender individuals due to homophobia were included in the analysis, but cannot be generalized to the transgender population.

On a separate measure, respondents were asked to respond to the statement, "I feel safe in my community in regard to my sexual orientation and/or gender identity." Response options ranged from 4 (*strongly agree*) to 0 (*strongly disagree*). Another question addressed housing instability and discrimination due to sexual orientation or gender identity. Respondents were asked to report if they "currently," "in the past," or "never" experienced housing instability or discrimination.

Mental health. The Patient Health Questionaire-2 (PHQ-2) was used to measure depression. The PHQ-2 comprises the first two items from the full depression scale, the PHQ-9. The stem question is, "Over the past two weeks, how often have you been bothered by any of the following problems?" The two items are "little interest or pleasure in doing things" and "feeling down, depressed, or hopeless." Answers were given on a scale ranging from 0 (*not at all*), 1 (*several days*), 2 (*more than half the days*), to 3 (*nearly every day*). The PHQ-2 score can range from zero to six. Previous findings support that a PHQ-2 cutoff score of ≥ 3 has the best tradeoff between sensitivity and specificity (Kroenke, Spitzer, & Williams, 2003; Löwe, Kroenke, & Gräfe,

2005). Therefore the responses were categorized as probable depression (score = 3–6) or no probable depression (score = 0–2).

After a comprehensive assessment, Löwe et al. (2005) established the reliability, construct and criterion validity, and sensitivity to change of the PHQ-2. Löwe et al. (2005) concluded that the PHQ-2 is a reliable (α = .83) and valid tool to assess depression severity, and diagnosis. Kroenke et al. (2003) also concluded that the construct and criterion validity of the PHQ-2 make it an attractive measure for depression screening. Li, Friedman, Conwell, and Fiscella (2007) found the PHQ-2 to be a valid screening tool for major depression in older people.

The Revised UCLA (University of California, Los Angeles) Loneliness Scale (R-UCLA) is a 20-item questionnaire that measures general feelings of isolation, dissatisfaction with social interactions, and loneliness (Russell, Peplau, & Cutrona, 1980). The R-UCLA is known as the most frequently used measure of loneliness (Cacioppo, Hughes, Waite, Hawkley, & Thisted, 2006). For this study, a three-item version of R-UCLA was used to measure loneliness. The three items included, "How often do you feel that you lack companionship?," "How often do you feel left out?," and "How often do you feel isolated from others?" Answers were given on a 3-point scale ranging from 1 (*hardly ever*), 2 (*sometimes*), to 3 (*often*). Responses to this scale were summed, with higher scores indicating greater loneliness (Hughes, Waite, Hawkley, & Cacioppo, 2004). The three-item R-UCLA score can range from three to nine. Hughes et al. found a strong correlation between the three-item R-UCLA and the full 20-item R-UCLA Loneliness Scale. The Cronbach's alpha for the three-item R-UCLA is .73 (Hughes et al., 2004).

Respondents

A total of 473 respondents completed the survey, ranging in age from 18 to 79 years old. Six respondents were not included in the final sample due to their identified zip code being outside Missouri or the greater metropolitan area of St. Louis. Another eight respondents were dropped from the sample because they did not self-identify as LGBT. A final sample of N = 459 was obtained. For the purposes of this study, we conducted an independent analysis of the data on LGBT adults over the age of 50 (N = 151). Respondents included in the final sample ranged in age from 50 to 79 years old. The sample was further divided into two groups, the Baby Boomers and the Silent generation based on age. Baby Boomers (n = 118) ranged in age from 50 to 64 years old, and the Silent generation (n = 33) ranged in age from 65 to 79 years old.

The needs assessment focused on the greater metropolitan area of St. Louis, which encompasses not only St. Louis City and St. Louis County, but geographic areas west and east of the Mississippi River, including the Missouri counties of St. Charles, Franklin, Jefferson, and six counties in

Illinois including Bond, Clinton, Madison, Monroe, St. Clair, and Washington. This geographic service region is diverse ranging from urban, suburban, and rural communities and is served by three Area Agencies on Aging. St. Louis City is viewed as the LGBT cultural and social center with many of the LGBT-friendly nonprofit organizations and businesses operating within the city of St. Louis. A concerted effort was made to collect surveys from across this diverse region, with the results forming the first regionally based study regarding LGBT older adults.

RESULTS

Demographics

The majority of respondents were from St. Louis City (37%) and St. Louis County (32%). Twelve percent of respondents were from other metropolitan Missouri counties and 10% of respondents were from Illinois counties in the greater metropolitan area of St. Louis. Three respondents (2%) were from Reynolds, Lincoln, and Camden counties in rural Missouri. These respondents were included in the sample, as SAGE would provide services to these respondents if needed. The county of eleven (7%) respondents was not known; it was assumed that these respondents were from the greater metropolitan area of St. Louis and therefore were included in the sample.

Table 1 outlines the proportions of the total sample and depicts the demographic characteristics of the Baby Boom generation and Silent generation within the sample. Of the 151 respondents, 47.7% identified as male, 45.7% as female, 0.6% as female-to-male transgender, and 3.3% as male-to-female transgender. Two respondents fell outside of these categorizations, with one respondent identifying as "butch lesbian" and another as "gender agnostic." Forty-nine percent of respondents exclusively identified as gay, 36.4% as lesbian, 7.3% as bisexual, and 7.3% identified as multiple labels including gay, lesbian, bisexual, queer, or other. The sample was predominantly Caucasian (90.1%), with an under-representation of African Americans (1.3%), Asians (0.7%), and individuals who identified as more than one race (2.6%). Three respondents identified as exclusively American Indian (2.0%) and three respondents fell outside of these categories with two respondents identifying as Jewish (1.3%) and one as American (0.7%).

As seen in Table 1, the average age of Baby Boomers in the sample was 55.9 ($SD = 4.3$), and the average age of Silents was 70.9 ($SD = 4.7$). Seven of the eight gender nonconforming respondents were members of the Baby Boom generation. The majority of respondents were highly educated. Close to 43% of Baby Boomers (42.7%) and 48.5% of Silents reported having an advanced degree, whereas the highest level of education reported by 11.1% of Baby Boomers and 12.1% of Silents was high school. Although the

TABLE 1 Demographic Characteristics of Baby Boomers and the Silent Generation From the 2010 Greater St. Louis Lesbian, Gay, Bisexual, and Transgender Health and Human Services Needs Assessment

Variable	Total Sample (*N* = 151) *n* (%)	Baby Boomers (*n* = 118) *n* (%)	Silent Generation (*n* = 33) *n* (%)
Age			
M	59.2	55.9	70.9
SD	7.6	4.3	4.7
Gender identity			
Female	69 (46.3)	57 (49.1)	12 (36.4)
Male	72 (48.3)	52 (44.8)	20 (60.6)
Male-to-female	5 (3.4)	4 (3.5)	1 (3.0)
Female-to-male	1 (0.7)	1 (0.9)	0 (0.0)
Other	2 (1.3)	2 (1.7)	0 (0.0)
Sexual orientation			
Lesbian	55 (36.4)	45 (38.1)	10 (30.3)
Gay	74 (49.0)	56 (47.5)	18 (54.5)
Bisexual	11 (7.3)	10 (8.5)	1 (3.0)
Multiple labels	11 (7.3)	7 (5.9)	4 (12.1)
Race/ethnicity			
American Indian	3 (2.0)	3 (2.6)	0 (0.0)
African American	2 (1.3)	2 (1.7)	0 (0.0)
Asian	1 (0.7)	1 (0.9)	0 (0.0)
Caucasian	136 (91.3)	104 (88.9)	32 (100.0)
Multiracial	4 (2.7)	4 (3.4)	0 (0.0)
Other	3 (2.0)	3 (2.5)	0 (0.0)
Have children			
Yes	60 (40.5)	42 (36.2)	18 (56.3)
No	88 (59.5)	74 (63.8)	14 (43.7)
Relationship status			
Not partnered	79 (54.5)	60 (53.1)	19 (59.4)
Same-sex partner	60 (41.4)	48 (42.5)	12 (37.5)
Different-sex partner	6 (4.1)	5 (4.4)	1 (3.1)
Household income			
<$10,000	8 (5.3)	6 (5.1)	2 (6.2)
$10,000–$20,000	16 (10.7)	13 (11.0)	3 (9.4)
$20,000–$35,000	34 (22.7)	22 (18.6)	12 (37.5)
$35,000–$50,000	19 (12.7)	16 (13.6)	3 (9.4)
$50,000–$75,000	33 (22.0)	29 (24.6)	4 (12.5)
$75,000–$100,000	22 (14.6)	15 (12.7)	7 (21.9)
$100,000+	18 (12.0)	17 (14.4)	1 (3.1)
Level of education			
Less than high school	1 (0.7)	1 (0.9)	0 (0.0)
High school/general equivalency diploma	17 (11.3)	13 (11.1)	4 (12.1)
College degree	66 (44.0)	53 (45.3)	13 (39.4)
Advanced degree	66 (44.0)	50 (42.7)	16 (48.5)
Employment			
Employed	83 (55.7)	74 (63.2)	9 (28.1)
Not employed	66 (44.3)	43 (36.8)	23 (71.9)

Note. The term *gay* is not particular to a gender.

sample lacked ethnic diversity, this is especially true for the Silent generation; all respondents from the Silent generation identified as Caucasian.

Silents were more likely to have children (56.3%) compared to Baby Boomers (36.2%), and more than 59% of Silents (59.4%) were not partnered compared to 53.1% of Baby Boomers, although these differences were not significant. In addition, 50.0% of female respondents reported having a child compared to 32.5% of male respondents ($\chi^2 = 4.70$, $p < .05$). Although not statistically significant, within the Baby Boom generation, 54.7% of female respondents were partnered, compared to 36.5% of male respondents. Within the Silent generation, 41.7% of female respondents were partnered compared to 36.8% of male respondents.

Respondents from both generations reported a wide variety of household incomes. Over 16% of Baby Boomers (16.2%) reported that their income does not cover their basic living expenses compared to 12.1% of Silents. Only one respondent (3.1%) from the Silent generation reported a household income over $100,000, compared to 14.4% of Baby Boomers. The largest proportion of Silents (37.5%) reported a household income from $20,000 to $35,000, while the largest proportion of Baby Boomers (24.6%) reported a household income from $50,000 to $75,000. It appears that Baby Boomers have a higher household income than members of the Silent generation— a difference likely influenced by a sizeable proportion of Baby Boomers remaining in the workforce compared to Silents. Although retirement status cannot be fully interpreted from the data, as expected, it appears that more Silents have entered retirement than Baby Boomers. More than 63% of Baby Boomers (63.2%) were employed compared to only 28.1% of Silents.

Barriers to Legal Services

Baby Boomers were significantly more likely to perceive barriers to legal services compared to members of the Silent generation ($t = 3.46$, $p < .001$). Close to 63% of Baby Boomers (62.8%) viewed restricted access to LGBT friendly attorneys as a barrier to legal services compared to 34.4% of Silents ($\chi^2 = 8.20$, $p < .01$). For both Baby Boomers and Silents, the greatest barrier to legal services was limited financial resources; however, significantly more Baby Boomers (78.3%) viewed this as a "major problem," "somewhat of a problem," or "slight problem" compared to Silents (54.5%; $\chi^2 = 7.30$, $p < .01$). Although not statistically significant, 42.9% of gender nonconforming respondents and 27.9% of female respondents reported that limited financial resources were a "major problem" in regard to accessing legal services, compared to 19.7% of male respondents.

A roughly equal proportion of Silents (45.5%) and Baby Boomers (46.9%) reported having a power of attorney for finances. There was also not a significant difference between generations in regard to power of attorney for health care. More than 63% of Silents (63.6%) and 61.1% of Baby Boomers reported having a power of attorney for health care. Over 30% of Silents (33.3%) and 19.5% of Baby Boomers reported having a trust.

Silents were more likely than Baby Boomers to have a will and living will in place. More than 75% of Silents (75.8%) reported having a will compared to 49.6% of Baby Boomers ($\chi^2 = 7.10$, $p < .01$). An equal proportion of Silents (75.8%) also reported having a living will, compared to 46.9% of Baby Boomers ($\chi^2 = 8.50$, $p < .01$). Although not a significant difference, 15.2% of Silents, compared to close to 30% of Baby Boomers (29.2%), had no legal documents in place.

Barriers to Health Care

The majority of Silents reported having Medicare or Medicaid (76.7%), whereas most Baby Boomers reported having health insurance through an employer (61.6%). All members of the Silent generation reported that they have some form of health insurance. However, over 10% of Baby Boomers (10.2%) did not have health insurance and of the uninsured Baby Boomers, 25.0% identified as gender nonconforming. The majority of Silents (90.9%) and Baby Boomers (83.9%) reported receiving primary health care from a private doctor as opposed to a community health center or an emergency room.

Overall Baby Boomers perceived more barriers related to health care access than Silents, $t(149) = 3.04$, $p < .001$. As seen in Figure 1, the most common cited barrier to health care for both LGBT Baby Boomers (70.3%) and the Silent generation (57.6%) was personal financial resources. However, 23.7% of Baby Boomers indicated that finances were a "major problem" compared to just 6.1% of Silents. Although not a significant relationship, more female (24.6%) and gender nonconforming (25.0%) respondents reported that personal finances were a "major problem," compared to 15.3% of male respondents.

More than 64% of Baby Boomers (64.3%) viewed a lack of support groups for LGBT people as a barrier to receiving needed services compared to 37.5% of Silents ($\chi^2 = 7.40$, $p < .01$). Both Baby Boomers (57.8%) and Silents (45.2%) felt that there were not enough adequately trained health professionals to deliver health care to LGBT people. More than 55% of Baby Boomers (55.2%) felt that there were not enough adequately trained and knowledgeable mental health professionals to help with their mental health issues, compared to only 12.1% of Silents ($\chi^2 = 19.20$, $p < .001$). Both members of the Silent generation (39.4%) and Baby Boomers (47.5%) were fearful that if medical professionals found out their sexual orientation or gender identity, they would be treated differently.

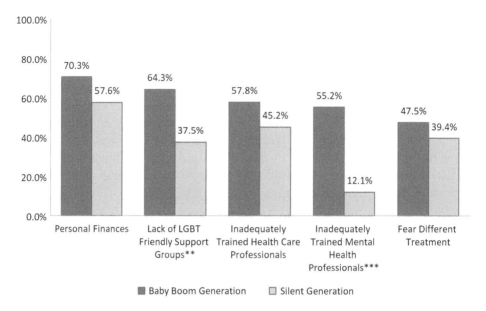

FIGURE 1 Perceived barriers to health care of lesbian, gay, bisexual, and transgender (LGBT) Baby Boomers and Silents. *Note.* Responses indicating a "major problem," "somewhat of a problem," or "very slight problem" were considered a "perceived barrier to health care." **$p < .01$. ***$p < .001$ (indicate significant differences between LGBT Baby Boomers and Silents).

LGBT Identity Disclosure

The majority of respondents reported a high level of LGBT identity disclosure. A significant correlation was found between age and LGBT identity disclosure; as age increased, level of disclosure decreased ($r = -.224$, $p < .01$). No significant gender differences were found. More than 80% of Silents (80.7%) and 72.8% of Baby Boomers *agreed* or *strongly agreed* that they were out to their health care provider. Close to 89% of LGBT Baby Boomers (88.9%) and 75.7% of Silents *agreed* or *strongly agreed* that they were out to their families. An even larger proportion of Baby Boomers (91.5%) and Silents (84.9%) *agreed* or *strongly agreed* that they were out to their friends. Twenty-five percent of Silents (25.0%) compared to 17.0% of Baby Boomers *disagreed* or *strongly disagreed* that they were out at work and 15 respondents (9.9%) did not answer the question. It is important to recognize that older respondents are more likely to be retired and may have reflected on their past work experience rendering this item different for the two groups.

In the past year, more than 36% of respondents from the Silent generation (36.4%) and 25.4% of Baby Boomers attended events specifically for LGBT people more than once per month. Only 12.1% of Silents and 6.8% of Baby Boomers have not attended an event specifically for the LGBT community in the past year. There was a significant difference between Baby

Boomers and Silents in regard to perceived use of an LGBT friendly health and human service provider list ($\chi^2 = 15.50$, $p < .001$). More than 60% of Baby Boomers (60.2%) reported that if a list of LGBT friendly health and human service providers were created, they would use this list "a lot," and an additional 22.0% reported they would "only choose providers from this list." In comparison, close to 40% of Silents (39.4%) believed they would use this list "a lot" and 12.1% would "only choose providers from this list."

Violence and Victimization

As depicted in Figure 2, 61.6% of respondents have experienced violence or victimization due to homophobia over their lifetime; however, only 17.2% of respondents have reported the incident. Over 24% of respondents (24.5%) have experienced solely verbal harassment, while the remaining 37.1% have endured neglect, physical assault, blackmail, property damage, or sexual assault due to homophobia. Overall, more than 58% of respondents (58.2%) have experienced verbal harassment due to homophobia. Male respondents reported experiencing significantly more types of violence and victimization due to homophobia than female respondents ($t = 2.64$, $p < .01$).

More than 26% of Baby Boomers (26.2%) compared to 9.1% of Silents reported that they *disagree* or *strongly disagree* with the statement, "I feel safe in my community in regard to my sexual orientation or gender identity" ($\chi^2 = 9.88$, $p < .05$). In addition, regardless of generational cohort, as experiences of different forms of violence and victimization increased, feelings of safety in community decreased ($r = -.230$, $p < .01$). There was also a significant correlation between feelings of safety in community and

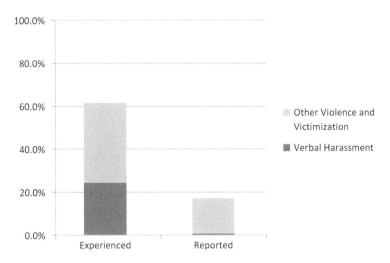

FIGURE 2 Total experienced violence and victimization due to homophobia.

LGBT identity disclosure. As feelings of safety in community increased, LGBT identity disclosure also increased ($r = .231, p < .01$).

Although a large proportion of Silents (40.0%) reported experiencing verbal harassment due to homophobia, more Baby Boomers (63.1%) reported being verbally harassed ($\chi^2 = 5.16, p < .05$). Although not a significant relationship, 18.6% of Baby Boomers have experienced housing discrimination due to their sexual orientation or gender identity compared to 3.1% of Silents. More than 21% of Baby Boomers (21.5%) and 19.2% of Silents have experienced property damage due to homophobia.

Over 21% of LGBT Baby Boomers (21.5%) have been physically assaulted, with 6.5% requiring medical attention. Similarly, 14.8% of Silents have been physically assaulted due to homophobia, with 7.7% requiring medical attention. In general, males were more likely to report experiencing physical assault due to homophobia than female respondents. Of the respondents physically assaulted due to homophobia, 81.5% were males and 18.5% were females ($\chi^2 = 13.10, p < .001$). Seven of the eight respondents who reported being sexually assaulted due to homophobia were also males. There were no significant differences between the cohorts on the continuous measure of violence and victimization. There was also not a significant correlation between experienced violence or victimization and LGBT identity disclosure.

Mental Health

More than 15% (i.e., 15.3%) of Baby Boomers and 12.1% of Silents had probable depression according to the PHQ-2. No significant differences were found between the Baby Boom and Silent generation on measures of loneliness and depression. Respondents with probable depression were significantly more likely to have endured different forms of violence and victimization due to homophobia ($t = 3.09, p < .01$). Respondents with probable depression were also significantly more likely to perceive more barriers to health care ($t = 3.35, p < .01$) and legal services ($t = 3.12, p < .01$).

The majority of Baby Boomers (58.5%) and Silents (65.7%) felt that they "sometimes" or "often" lack companionship. Twenty-two percent of Baby Boomers (22.0%) and 9.1% of Silents "often" feel isolated from others. A similar proportion of Baby Boomers (21.2%) and Silents (9.4%) "often" feel left out. Regardless of generation, as LGBT identity disclosure decreased, loneliness increased ($r = -.264, p < .01$). As loneliness increased, perceived barriers to health care ($r = .416, p < .001$) and legal services also increased ($r = .385, p < .001$). There was also a significant correlation between loneliness and experiencing different forms of violence and victimization due to homophobia ($r = .386, p < .001$). There was not a significant association between depression and relationship status; however, partnered respondents were significantly less likely to be lonely ($t = 7.12, p < .001$).

DISCUSSION

Many differences were found between Baby Boomers and members of the Silent generation from the Greater St. Louis LGBT Health and Human Services Needs Assessment. These findings indicate that Baby Boomers perceive more barriers to health care and legal services, have fewer legal documents in place, feel less safe in their communities, and have experienced an increased rate of verbal harassment compared to their predecessors. The findings also suggest that as age increases, level of LGBT identity disclosure decreases. It is proposed that a greater level of LGBT identity disclosure among Baby Boomers has brought opportunities for change, but also produced challenges.

Demographics

Demographic differences and similarities were found between the two generations in this study; these findings have both empirical and policy/program implications. Although not statistically significant, members of the Silent generation were more likely to have children than members of the Baby Boom generation. This could be due to major cultural shifts that occurred early in the lives of many Baby Boomers and later for members of the Silent generation—that is, Silents came of age during a time when adherence to the ethics and values of the dominate culture defined the character of an individual and conformity was expected (G. Williams, 2002). It might be said that hetero-conformity in young adulthood for members of the Silent generation involved establishing nuclear families, whereas members of the Baby Boom generation were allowed more flexibility in this regard.

The findings related to having children were both inconsistent and consistent with previous studies. The men and women of this sample were more likely to have children than reported in the first national community-based survey of LGBT adults over the age of 50 (Fredriksen-Goldsen et al., 2011). Compared to 40.5% of older LGBT adults in this study, researchers found that 25% of respondents had one or more children (Fredriksen-Goldsen et al., 2011). However, consistent with this study, Adelman, Gurevitch, de Vries, and Blando (2006) found that 28% of gay men and 57% of lesbians over the age of 65 have one or more children. In this study, female respondents (50.0%) were also more likely to report having a child compared to male respondents (32.5%).

Consistent with previous studies, close to one-half of the LGBT older adults in the sample were not partnered, and women were more likely to be partnered than men (Black, Gates, Sanders, & Taylor, 2000; Fredriksen-Goldsen et al., 2011; MetLife, 2006). A similar proportion of Silents and Baby Boomers were in a relationship; however, slightly more members of the Baby Boom generation (46.9%) were partnered compared to members of the Silent generation (40.6%). This slight difference could be due to age-related factors—that is, perhaps more members of the Silent generation have experienced the loss of a partner compared to members of the Baby Boom generation; however, this was not addressed in this study. Fredriksen-Goldsen et al. (2011) found that 27% of LGBT older adults have experienced the death of a partner. It is also worth noting that a significant proportion of gay men (MetLife, 2010) report never having had a partner; the experiences of singlehood were not addressed in this study and need to be fully explored.

Both Baby Boomers and Silents reported a wide variety of household incomes. Respondents from both generations were also highly educated comparable to the findings of Adelman et al. (2006). Corresponding with Fredriksen-Goldsen et al. (2011), 16% of LGBT older adults in this study had an annual household income of less than $20,000—a proportion that was consistent across the two generations. Similar to the general older adult population, the main concern of LGBT Baby Boomers is financial stability (MetLife, 2010; Orel, 2004). In this study, the number one barrier to health care and legal services for both Baby Boomers and Silents was personal financial resources. However, a larger proportion of Baby Boomers than Silents viewed financial resources as a problem. Members of the Silent generation are more likely to rely on fixed-benefit pension plans in retirement than members of the Baby Boom generation, which could influence differences in the perception of financial stability (Salkowitz, 2008).

In this study, all members of the Silent generation had health insurance, while 10.2% of Baby Boomers were uninsured. This finding is likely associated with the majority of Silents qualifying for (and receiving) Medicare. Consistent with previous findings, gender nonconforming respondents were more likely to be uninsured (Cahill et al., 2000; M. E. Williams & Freeman, 2007). Lack of health insurance coverage exacerbates the unique health challenges that transgendered individuals face. Training health care providers on these unique challenges is needed to help alleviate health disparities. Changes to the health care system are also necessary to promote equal access to health care for transgendered individuals.

Disclosure and Its Implications

Within the Baby Boom generation is the largest cohort of LGBT individuals who have had the opportunity to live their lives openly. In this study, as age increased, level of LGBT identity disclosure decreased. Baby Boomers were also more likely than Silents to have experienced verbal harassment due to homophobia. An association between earlier self-disclosure of sexual orientation and more experiences of victimization has also been documented (D'Augelli et al., 2001). It is possible that due to cultural shifts, Baby Boomers were more likely to disclose their LGBT identity at an earlier age, leading to more Baby Boomers experiencing verbal harassment than Silents.

Overall, Baby Boomers perceived significantly more barriers to health care than Silents. This difference could be attributed to the higher level of LGBT identity disclosure among Baby Boomers and therefore increased perception of negative reactions to their LGBT identity in health care settings. General cohort differences also may influence perception of barriers to health care and legal services. The Baby Boom generation is known to challenge restrictions and may have higher expectations than members of the Silent generation when accessing services (Hooyman & Kiyak, 2011).

In line with findings related to perceived barriers to health care, significantly more LGBT Baby Boomers perceived barriers to legal services as a problem compared to members of the Silent generation. This again could be related to a legitimate fear among Baby Boomers that they are more likely to face discrimination when accessing legal services due to a higher level of LGBT identity disclosure. LGBT Silents were also more likely to have a will and living will in place than LGBT Baby Boomers. Consistent with previous findings, close to one-half (53.1%) of Baby Boomers in this study reported not having a living will (MetLife, 2010). Having legal documents in place is especially important for partnered individuals within the LGBT community who do not have the same rights as their heterosexual counterparts. The creation of targeted programs to decrease barriers to legal services and assist LGBT Baby Boomers with legal document preparation is crucial.

Consistent with the role of minority stress, as defined by Meyer (2003), respondents with probable depression and increased loneliness were more likely to have endured different forms of violence and victimization due to homophobia. LGBT older adults are also less likely to seek supportive services, which in turn may leave them at risk for social isolation and depression (Butler, 2004; Cahill, 2000). The higher prevalence of verbal harassment experienced by LGBT Baby Boomers could also influence their increased perception of barriers to health care and legal services compared to Silents. For example, an experience of verbal harassment is likely to increase vigilance and the expectation that a similar incident will happen again (Meyer, 2003).

According to this study, 15% (15.3%) of Baby Boomers and 12.1% of Silents are depressed. Practitioners and researchers agree that depression is key risk factors of suicide (Institute of Medicine, 2002). In the United States and across the world, suicide rates generally increase with age, making older adults an at risk population (World Health Organization, 2002). This increased risk has been attributed to untreated depression, which can be exacerbated by the many losses that can accompany later life (Kent, 2010). A relationship between sexual minority status and elevated rates of suicidal behavior has also been observed across the life course (Mathy, 2002). Thus, sexual minority status and increased age are important risk factors for adverse mental health outcomes among LGBT older adults and should be explored further in future research.

Baby Boomers were also significantly less likely than Silents to feel safe in their community based on their sexual orientation or gender identity. A significant correlation was also found between feelings of safety in community and experiences of different types of violence and victimization. As experiences of different forms of violence and victimization increased, feelings of safety in community decreased. Since Baby Boomers were significantly more likely to experience verbal harassment and not feel safe in their community compared to Silents, it can be inferred that these experiences influence feelings of safety for LGBT Baby Boomers.

Based on the previous discussion, it was surprising to find that as LGBT identity disclosure increased, feelings of safety in community also increased. One explanation is that LGBT individuals with higher levels of identity disclosure are more likely to live in communities that are accepting of their identity. It is also possible that living in an open and inclusive community increases the likelihood of LGBT identity disclosure.

Close to 62% of respondents (61.6%) have experienced violence or victimization due to homophobia over their lifetime, yet only 17.2% of respondents have reported the incident. Avenues for LGBT individuals to report violence or victimization are limited due to a lack of non-discrimination policies and procedures inclusive of sexual orientation and gender identity. Without these mechanisms in place, LGBT individuals may well continue to be victimized with few, if any, safe options to report the incident.

Living in a world that stigmatizes LGBT individuals, the findings of this study support the perspective that LGBT identity disclosure brings both risk and opportunity. It can be deduced that disclosure of LGBT identity can positively affect mental wellbeing while also increasing stress on LGBT individuals due to incongruence between their needs and societal structures (D'Augelli & Grossman, 2001). Human service practitioners and policy makers must collaborate and advocate for non-discrimination policies inclusive of sexual orientation and gender identity to reduce the incongruence between the needs of LGBT individuals and heteronormative structures that are in place.

Limitations and Implications

This study had several limitations which should be considered. First, convenience and snowball sampling techniques were used. LGBT individuals were recruited through local LGBT organization Web sites, newsletters, listservs, and social media outlets. Therefore, respondents most likely had a higher level of LGBT identity disclosure and were more active in the LGBT community compared to the general older LGBT population.

The sample also over-represented individuals easily accessible by online surveys including younger older adults, highly educated individuals, and Caucasian respondents. A small number of bisexual and gender nonconforming respondents were included in the sample. Due to these sample limitations, the results of this study cannot be generalized to the entire population of LGBT older adults in the St. Louis region.

The measure of overall LGBT identity disclosure had 16 respondents with missing data. This measure was created by summing four Likert scale items in relation to family, friends, health care, and work. If a respondent did not answer one of these four items, the LGBT disclosure variable was coded as missing. Otherwise a respondent's score could be misrepresented as a lower value that may not reflect their level of LGBT identity disclosure. After further examination it was determined that 13 respondents were only missing data in relation to LGBT disclosure at work, and nine of these respondents were over the age of 60. This suggests that respondents might have intentionally skipped this question because they are retired, and therefore the question did not apply. It is important to carefully consider each question when developing or implementing a survey instrument to reduce the potential for missing data when targeting an older population. There also were not questions in the needs assessment that asked specifically about retirement or health status. These limitations should be considered when developing future needs assessments. Collecting information related to retirement and health status is essential to better understanding the needs of LGBT older adults.

Demographic variations and sample size differences between the Baby Boom generation and the Silent generation could also have influenced the results. For instance, almost all gender nonconforming respondents were members of the Baby Boom generation and all members of the Silent generation identified as Caucasian. Despite these drawbacks, this study contributed to present knowledge of the needs of LGBT older adults and helps support programs and services specific to this population.

For example, based on the findings of this study, SAGE Metro St. Louis has made it a priority to build relationships with older adult service organizations to help ensure safe and welcoming service provision for LGBT older adults. To decrease barriers to health care, SAGE partnered with the Long-Term Care Ombudsman Program to train nursing home staff and administrators on the unique needs of LGBT older adults. SAGE also became a certified trainer for the National Resource Center on LGBT Aging cultural competence training, a national effort to help increase overall competency when serving LGBT older adults.

The findings of the Greater St. Louis LGBT Health and Human Services Needs Assessment have been used to support requests for funding programs and services to meet the needs of LGBT older adults. Researchers of this study determined that the majority of Baby Boomers (58.5%) and Silents (65.7%) felt that they "sometimes" or "often" lack companionship; as a result, SAGE has established a friendly visitor program to reach homebound LGBT older adults who are at risk for loneliness and isolation.

Preliminary results from this study were presented at a health care provider forum in the summer of 2011. The aim of the forum was to begin community dialogue regarding the issues of LGBT health access and disparities. Following this forum, SAGE and PROMO, the Missouri Statewide equality organization, received funding from the Missouri Foundation for Health for a planning grant to address LGBT health disparities in Missouri. In addition, to address the perceived lack of adequately trained mental health professionals, SAGE joined an advisory council designed to increase awareness and training of mental health professionals and expand outreach to the LGBT community.

The findings of this study have helped SAGE understand the needs and perspectives of the current cohort of LGBT older adults and anticipate upcoming changes with the appearance of the Baby Boom generation. It is evident that LGBT Silents have faced obstacles throughout their lives living in a world with incongruence between their needs and societal structures. Due to higher levels of LGBT identity disclosure among Baby Boomers, this incongruence has shifted. LGBT Baby Boomers are more fearful when accessing services and have experienced an increased rate of verbal harassment. This shift will bring challenges and opportunities for organizations like SAGE working to enhance the lives of LGBT older adults. Ongoing efforts are needed to build awareness, advance practice, and create policies that improve the lives of LGBT individuals across the life course.

REFERENCES

Adelman, M., Gurevitch, J., de Vries, B., & Blando, J. A. (2006). Community building and research in the LGBT aging population. In D. Kimmel, T. Rose, & S. David (Eds.), *Lesbian, gay, bisexual, and transgender aging* (pp. 1–19). New York, NY: Columbia University Press.

American Psychiatric Association. (1973, December 15). *Press release*. Washington, DC: Author.

Anetzberger, G. J., Ishler, K. J., Mostade, J., & Blair, M. (2004). Gray and gay: A community dialogue on the issues and concerns of older gays and lesbians. *Journal of Gay & Lesbian Social Services, 17*(1), 23–41.

Balsam, K. F., Rothblum, E. D., & Beauchaine, T. P. (2005). Victimization over the lifespan: A comparison of lesbian, gay, bisexual, and heterosexual siblings. *Journal of Consulting and Clinical Psychology, 73*, 477–487.

Black, D., Gates, G., Sanders, S., & Taylor, L. (2000). Demographics of the gay and lesbian population in the United States: Evidence from available systematic data sources. *Demography, 32*, 139–154.

Blando, J. A. (2001). Twice hidden: Older gay and lesbian couples, friends, and intimacy. *Generations, 25*(2), 87–89.

Brotman, S., Ryan, B., & Cormier, R. (2003). The health and social service needs of gay and lesbian elders and their families in Canada. *Gerontologist, 43*, 192–202.

Butler, S. (2004). Gay, lesbian, bisexual, and transgender (GLBT) elders: The challenges and resilience of this marginalized group. *Journal of Human Behavior in the Social Environment*, 9(4), 25–44.

Cacioppo, J. T., Hughes, M. E., Waite, L. J., Hawkley, L. C., & Thisted, R. (2006). Loneliness as a specific risk factor for depressive symptoms: Cross-sectional and longitudinal analyses. *Psychology and Aging*, 21(1), 140–151.

Cahill, S. (2002). Long term care issues affecting gay, lesbian, bisexual and transgender elders. *Geriatric Care Management Journal*, 12(3), 4–8.

Cahill, S., South, K., & Spade, J. (2000). *Outing age public policy issues affecting gay, lesbian, bisexual and transgender elders*. New York, NY: Public Policy Institute of the National Gay and Lesbian Task Force.

Centers for Disease Control and Prevention. (2009). *Audience insights: Communicating to the responsible generation*. Atlanta, GA: Author.

Cochran, S. D., & Mays, V. M. (2000). Relation between psychiatric syndromes and behaviorally defined sexual orientation in a sample of the US population. *American Journal of Epidemiology*, 151, 516–523.

Corliss, H. L., Cochran, S. D., & Mays, V. M. (2002). Reports of parental maltreatment during childhood in a United States population-based survey of homosexual, bisexual, and heterosexual adults. *Child Abuse & Neglect*, 26, 1165–1178.

D'Augelli, A. R., & Grossman, A. H. (2001). Disclosure of sexual orientation, victimization, and mental health among lesbian, gay, and bisexual older adults. *Journal of Interpersonal Violence*, 16, 1008–1027.

D'Augelli, A. R., Grossman, A. H., Hershberger, S. L., & O'Connell, T. S. (2001). Aspects of mental health among older lesbian, gay, and bisexual adults. *Aging and Mental Health*, 5, 149–158.

D'Augelli, A. R., Hershberger, S. L., & Pilkington, N. W. (1998). Lesbian, gay, and bisexual youths and their families: Disclosure of sexual orientation and its consequences. *American Journal of Orthopsychiatry*, 68, 361–371.

Dychtwald, K. (2000). *Age power: How the 21st century will be ruled by the new old*. New York, NY: Putnam.

Egri, C. P., & Ralston, D. A. (2004). Generation cohorts and personal values: A comparison of China and the United States. *Organization Science*, 15, 210–220.

Frazer, M. S. (2009). *LGBT Health and Human Services needs in New York state*. Albany, NY: Empire State Pride Agenda Foundation. Retrieved from http://www.prideagenda.org/Portals/0/pdfs/LGBT%20Health%20and%20Human%20Services%20Needs%20in%20New%20York%20State.pdf

Fredriksen-Goldsen, K. I., Kim, H., Emlet, C. A., Muraco, A., Erosheva, E. A., Hoy-Ellis, C. P., . . . Petry, H. (2011). *The aging and health report: Disparities and resilience among lesbian, gay, bisexual, and transgender older adults*. Seattle, WA: Institute for Multigenerational Health. Retrieved from http://caringandaging.org/wordpress/wp-content/uploads/2011/05/Full-Report-FINAL-11-16-11.pdf

Friedman, R. C. (1999). Homosexuality, psychopathology, and suicidality. *Archives of General Psychiatry*, 56, 887–888.

Gilman, S. E., Cochran, S. D., Mays, V. M., Hughes, M., Ostrow, D., & Kessler, R. C. (2001). Risks of psychiatric disorders among individuals reporting same-sex sexual partners in the National Comorbidity Survey. *American Journal of Public Health, 91*, 933–939.

Grant, J. M. (2010). *Outing Age 2010: Public policy issues affecting lesbian, gay, bisexual, and transgender elders*. Washington, DC: National Gay and Lesbian Task Force Policy Institute. Retrieved from http://www.thetaskforce.org/downloads/reports/reports/outingage_final.pdf

Grossman, A. H., D'Augelli, A. R., & O'Connell, T. S. (2001). Being lesbian, gay, bisexual, and sixty or older in North America. *Journal of Gay & Lesbian Social Services, 13*(4), 23–40.

Hash, K. M., & Cramer, E. P. (2003). Empowering gay and lesbian caregivers and uncovering their unique experiences through the use of qualitative methods. *Journal of Gay & Lesbian Social Services, 15*(1/2), 47–63.

Hooyman, N. R., & Kiyak, H. A. (2011). *Social gerontology: A multidisciplinary perspective* (9th ed.). Boston, MA: Allyn & Bacon.

Hughes, M. E., Waite, L. J., Hawkley, L. C., & Cacioppo, J. T. (2004). A short scale for measuring loneliness in large surveys: Results from two population-based studies. *Research on Aging, 26*, 655–672.

Institute of Medicine. (2002). *Reducing suicide: A national imperative*. Washington, DC: National Academies Press.

Institute of Medicine. (2011). *The health of lesbian, gay, bisexual, and transgender people: Building a foundation for better understanding*. Washington, DC: National Academies Press.

Johnson, R. W., Butrica, B. A., & Mommaerts, C. (2010). *Work and retirement patterns for the G.I. generation, silent generation, and early boomers: Thirty years of change (Retirement Policy Program)*. Washington, DC: Urban Institute.

Kent, M. M. (2010). *In U.S. Who is at greatest risk for suicide?* Washington, DC: Population Reference Bureau. Retrieved from http://www.prb.org/Publications/Articles/2010/suicides.aspx

Kimmel, D., Rose, T., Orel, N., & Greene, B. (2006). Historical context for research on lesbian, gay, bisexual, and transgender aging. In D. Kimmel, T. Rose, & S. David (Eds.), *Lesbian, gay, bisexual, and transgender aging* (pp. 1–19). New York, NY: Columbia University Press.

King, S., & Dabelko-Schoeny, H. (2009). "Quite frankly, I have doubts about remaining": Aging-in-place and health care access for rural midlife and older lesbian, gay and bisexual individuals. *Journal of LGBT Health Research, 5*, 10–21.

Kroenke, K., Spitzer, R. L., & Williams, J. B. (2003). The Patient Health Questionnaire-2: Validity of a two item depression screener. *Medical Care, 41*, 1284–1292.

Kuyper, L., & Fokkema, T. (2010). Loneliness among older lesbian, gay, and bisexual adults: The role of stress. *Archives of Sexual Behavior, 39*, 1171–1180.

Li, C., Friedman, B., Conwell, Y., & Fiscella, K. (2007). Validity of the Patient Health Questionnaire 2 (PHQ-2) in identifying major depression in older people. *Journal of the American Geriatrics Society, 55*, 596–602.

Lombardi, E. L., Wilchins, R. A., Priesing, D., & Malouf, D. (2002). Gender violence: Transgender experiences with violence and discrimination. *Journal of Homosexuality, 42*(1), 89–101.

Löwe, B., Kroenke, K., & Gräfe, K. (2005). Detecting and monitoring depression with a two-item questionnaire (PHQ–2). *Journal of Psychosomatic Research, 58,* 163–171.

Maccio, E. M., & Doueck, H. J. (2002). Meeting the needs of the gay and lesbian community: Outcomes in the human services. *Journal of Gay & Lesbian Social Services, 14*(4), 55–73.

Mathy, R. M. (2002). Suicidality and sexual orientation in five continents: Asia, Australia, Europe, North America, and South America. *International Journal of Sexuality and Gender Studies, 7,* 215–225.

MetLife Mature Market Institute, Lesbian and Gay Aging Issues Network of the American Society on Aging (2010). Out and aging: The MetLife study of lesbian and gay baby boomers. *Journal of GLBT Family Studies, 6,* 40–57.

MetLife Mature Market Institute. (2006). *Out and aging: The MetLife study of lesbian and gay baby boomers.* Westport, CT: Author.

Meyer, I. H. (2003). Prejudice, social stress, and mental health in lesbian, gay, and bisexual populations: Conceptual issues and research evidence. *American Psychological Association, 129,* 674–697.

Orel, N. A. (2004). Gay, lesbian, and bisexual elders: Expressed needs and concerns across focus groups. *Journal of Gerontological Social Work, 43*(2/3), 57–77.

Phillips, J., & Marks, G. (2006). Coming out, coming in: How do dominant discourses around aged care facilities take into account the identities and needs of aging lesbians? *Gay and Lesbian Issues and Psychology Review, 2*(2), 67–76.

Reingold, D., & Burros, N. (2004). Sexuality in the nursing home. *Journal of Gerontological Social Work, 43*(2/3), 175–186.

Russell, D., Peplau, L. A., & Cutrona, C. E. (1980). The revised UCLA Loneliness Scale: Concurrent and discriminant validity evidence. *Journal of Personality and Social Psychology, 39,* 472–480.

Salkowitz, R. (2008). *Generation blend: Managing across the technology age gap.* Hoboken, NJ: Wiley.

Sandfort, T. G., de Graaf, R., Bijl, R. V., & Schnabel, P. (2001). Same-sex sexual behavior and psychiatric disorders: Findings from the Netherlands Mental Health Survey and Incidence Study (NEMESIS). *Archives of General Psychiatry, 58,* 85–91.

Shankle, M. D., Maxwell, C. A., Katzman, E. S., & Landers, S. (2003). An invisible population: Older lesbian, gay, bisexual, and transgender individuals. *Clinical Research & Regulatory Affairs, 20,* 159–182.

Steinsvåg, B. A., Sandkjaer, B., & Størksen, I. (2004). Assessing health and social services needs in the GLB population: The Norwegian experience. *Journal of Gay & Lesbian Social Services, 16,* 147–163.

U.S. Census Bureau. (2010). *American Community Survey 2006–2010.* Washington, DC: Author. Retrieved from http://www.census.gov/acs/www/

U.S. Census Bureau. (2011). *Population profile of the United States.* Washington, DC: Author. Retrieved from http://csrd.asu.edu/sites/default/files/pdf/Population%20Profile%20of%20the%20United%20States.pdf

Ward, R., Vass, A. A., Aggarwal, N., Garfield, C., & Cybyk, B. (2005). A kiss is still a kiss? The construction of sexuality in dementia care. *Dementia, 4*(1), 49–72.

Williams, G. (2002). *Multi-generational marketing for non-profits*. Winnipeg, Manitoba, Canada: Planned Legacy. Retrieved from http://www.plannedlegacy. com/newsletter/fall2002/generationalmarketing.html

Williams, M. E., & Freeman, P. A. (2007). Transgender health: Implications for aging and caregiving. *Journal of Gay & Lesbian Social Services*, *18*, 93–108.

World Health Organization. (2002). *World report on violence and health*. Geneva, Switzerland: Author.

The Younger Generation. (1951, November 5). *Time Magazine*. Retrieved from http://www.time.com/time/subscriber/article/0,33009,856950,00.html

Aging Out in the Desert: Disclosure, Acceptance, and Service Use Among Midlife and Older Lesbians and Gay Men

AARON T. GARDNER, MA

County of Riverside Department of Public Health, Riverside, California, USA

BRIAN de VRIES, PhD

Gerontology Program, San Francisco State University, San Francisco, California, USA

DANYTE S. MOCKUS, PhD, MPH

County of Riverside Department of Public Health, Riverside, California, USA

Lesbian, gay, bisexual, and transgender (LGBT) persons in the county of Riverside, CA and in the Palm Springs/Coachella Valley area, in particular, responded to a questionnaire addressing concerns about identity disclosure and comfort accessing social services. Distributed at a Pride festival, as well as through religious, social, and service agencies, the final sample for analysis of 502 comprised 401 (80%) gay men and 101 (20%) lesbians in 4 groups: < 50 years of age (18%), 50 to 59 (26%), 60 to 69 (36%), and over 70 (20%). Results reveal that almost one-third of midlife and older gay men and lesbians maintain some fear of openly disclosing their sexual orientation. Along comparable lines with similar proportions, older gay men and lesbians maintain some discomfort in their use of older adult social services, even as the majority reports that they would feel more comfortable accessing LGBT-friendly identified services and programs. In both cases, lesbians reported greater fear and discomfort than did gay men; older gay men and lesbians reported that they would be less comfortable accessing LGBT-identified services and programs than did younger gay men and lesbians. These data support prior research on the

The authors thank the following for their assistance in the preparation of this article: Carolyn Lieber, Marshare Penny, Kevin Meconis, Ed Walsh, Lael Gardner-Stalnaker, and the Riverside County Office on Aging Planning Unit.

apprehension of LGBT elders in accessing care, the crucial role of acceptance, with some suggestions of how social services might better prepare to address these needs.

For lesbian, gay, bisexual, and transgender (LGBT) persons, disclosure (i.e., "coming out") represents the dynamic balance of the perceived safety (physical, emotional, and beyond) of a social setting and the experience or anticipated comfort and authenticity of the LGBT person in that setting. Such appraisals of safety and comfort are unfortunately routine components of social interactions for LGBT persons, part of the lifelong process of coming out (de Vries & Blando, 2004) with potential and significant costs to health and wellbeing (e.g., Meyer, 2003). Such appraisals ultimately serve as the context within which subsequent interactions take place (or not). To better understand some of these factors (e.g., level of comfort or fear and factors that signal organization/setting safety and potential use), a survey was administered by the Office on Aging in Riverside County in 2008. The results of this survey are reported later and highlight areas of concerns of lesbian and gay older adults; implications and courses of action are suggested.

BACKGROUND

Having come of age before the modern LGBT civil rights movement that is commonly believed to have begun with Stonewall in 1969, many of the LGBT elders of today have lived a large part of their lives in an environment characterized by hostility, neglect, and misunderstanding (Cahill, South, & Spade, 2000). These life experiences can have profound effects including, for example, the extent to which many of those in the older cohorts of LGBT populations are "out," particularly in healthcare and related settings, and their associated experiences of comfort and fear.

Age has been found to be associated with levels of disclosure. For example, Rawls (2004) reanalyzed data from the Urban Men's Health Study, a probabilistic sample of men who have sex with men; he reported that disclosure decreased across the increasing age groups he studied: 50 to 59 years, 60 to 69 years, and 70 years and older. In this analysis, about 5% of the men in this sample had *never* told someone that they were gay or bisexual. Comparably, Gates (2010) analyzed data from the General Social Survey and reported that, relative to those under age 30, gay men, lesbians, and bisexual women and men over the age of 55 were more likely to be closeted—83% more likely by his calculations! Across all age groups, nearly 13% of respondents had never come out to anyone.

Examining this from another perspective, in the Still Out, Still Aging: The MetLife study of LGBT boomers (with respondents aged 45–64; MetLife, 2010), about three-fourths of gay men and lesbians reported that they were completely out; the comparable percentages for transgender and bisexual male and female boomers were significantly lower at 39% and 16%, respectively. Respondents were also asked about the extent to which they were "guarded" about their sexual orientation or gender identity—a way of conceptualizing forms of non-disclosure. Almost 30% were not guarded with anyone; about one-fourth of respondents were guarded with neighbors and slightly less with other family. Bisexual boomers were more guarded than were gay men, lesbians, or transgender person—almost twice as many in some cases. Approximately 12% of gay men and lesbians were guarded with their health care provider—more than twice as many bisexual and transgender women and men reported being guarded (or not out).

Such issues of disclosure are undoubtedly a factor in the growing body of research that finds that many LGBT elders do not access medical care with the same frequency as their heterosexual counterparts (Movement Advancement Project, 2010). The anticipated stigma and discrimination (e.g., MetLife, 2010) may lead to deferred or delayed health care utilization with missed opportunities for preventive intervention (Bonvicini & Perlin, 2003). Sadly, these anticipated experiences have roots in the lived experiences of other LGBT elders. Brotman, Ryan, and Cornier (2003), for example, found that discrimination continues to be present in aging health care and social services. They report that, at best, there is a pervasive ignorance about gay and lesbian elders and their unique needs in the elder care network; at worst, there is ongoing hostility. A 2009 nationwide survey of 4,916 LGBT and HIV-positive individuals conducted by Lambda Legal, almost 8% of LGB, and 27% of transgender respondents reported being refused necessary health care because of their sexual orientation or gender nonconformity (Lambda Legal, 2010).

Parallels to such dramatic findings exist in studies describing the use of other services and agencies. In a study of readiness to serve, Knochel, Croghan, Moone, and Quam (2010) found that more than one-half of the Area Agencies on Aging (AAA) surveyed had not offered or funded any LGBT aging training to staff and very few were providing any LGBT aging outreach. These (in)actions have not gone unnoticed by LGBT older adults. The National Resource Center on LGBT Aging (2010) noted that many older LGBT adults are apprehensive of aging service providers for fear of discrimination and harassment should their sexual orientation or gender identity become known. Such experiences have either led LGBT adults away from such agencies—or back to the closet in order to participate in the agency programs or to access the needed services.

Together, these findings suggest the impact of perceived acceptance on accessing services needed by the aging LGBT population. It is critical to know the percentages of out LGBT persons across various environments and their level of comfort in accessing services. If agencies are to succeed in reaching out to these populations, such information is a prerequisite for the effective presentation and delivery of services.

METHOD

In 2007, the Riverside County Office on Aging (RCOA) sought to understand the perceptions and attitudes of the elder LGBT community in Riverside County, with a particular emphasis on Palm Springs. In the 2010 U.S. Census, Riverside County had the fourth largest proportion of same-sex senior couples in California; Palm Springs had the highest percentage of same-sex couples (Gates & Cooke, 2011). In addition, Riverside County ranked ninth in the nation in total number of same-sex couples that included a partner over 65 years old and eighth in the nation for couples that included a partner over 55 (Romero, Rosky, Badgett, Lee, & Gates, 2008). This is likely an undercount given the tremendous growth Riverside County has experienced over the past decade, but still indicates the significant presence and relevance of LGBT older adults in this county and region.

To better understand their experiences, a brief survey was created, funded by the county Office on Aging and informed by preliminary interviews and focus groups, for distribution at public gatherings. Attempting to balance anticipated response rates with ease of sample access, the short survey addressed sexual orientation and gender identity and included demographic questions about age (in decades from under 20 to over 90) and race/ethnicity (in distinct categories). Given the nature of the Palm Springs/Coachella Valley area as a destination resort community for LGBT persons, and older persons in particular, questions on the survey asked about residency status in the desert communities and the importance of LGBT-acceptance in residency or visiting decisions (e.g., the importance of sexual orientation/gender identity acceptance by a community/area in choosing a place to live or visit, with responses ranging from *very important* to *not important*).

Questions were posed addressing levels of comfort in use of services directed to older adults. These included a question addressing the perceived level of discomfort using social services (e.g., home-delivered meals, transportation, care management, caregiver support, respite, and senior employment), with responses of *yes, maybe,* and *no.* Specific questions were included asking if respondents would be more comfortable using the services of agencies identified as "gay or LGBT friendly" (including the posting of the Rainbow Flag; with responses of *comfortable, somewhat comfortable,* or *no difference*), and if the inclusion of gay/lesbian couples on promotional materials would influence decisions to use social services (with responses of *yes, maybe,* or *no*). Questions also asked if respondents participated in any LGBT organizations (and, if so, which ones) and if respondents participated in any senior social organizations (and, if so, which ones). To address comfort with disclosure, a question was posed inquiring if the respondent feared openly identifying as an LGBT person (with response categories being *yes, somewhat,* or *no*); a second question asked about the importance of feeling accepted as an LGBT person in the community in which one lives (with responses of *very, somewhat,* or *not important*). Space was provided for respondents to add any issues, concerns or services related to older LGBT individuals that they would like to see considered in the strategic planning of the County Office on Aging.

Questionnaires were initially distributed at the 2007 Palm Springs Pride weekend events. Subsequent surveys were distributed through contacts with lesbian and gay social and religious organizations. In partnership with the Golden Rainbow Senior Center (now a SAGE [Services and Advocacy for GLBT Elders] affiliate and part of The Center, a broader organization supporting the LGBT community more holistically), a wider sampling of the LGBT community was achieved. Beyond the senior center participants themselves, the questionnaire was disseminated in a variety of social and religious organizations. It is worth remembering that surveys were collected in and around the Palm Springs area at gay friendly venues and, hence, the extent to which this sample may be considered representative of the Riverside County LGBT population as a whole is questioned.

RESULTS

The total sample of 569 disproportionately comprised gay men: 401 (70%) respondents identified as gay male, and 101 (18%) identified as lesbian. The remainder identified as bisexual male (14; 2%) or bisexual female (6; 1%). Only 1 person identified as male-to-female transgender, 6 persons identified as straight male, and 40 persons identified as straight female. There was a broad range of ages of the respondents, as described in Table 1. The majority of respondents was Caucasian/White (87%) and came from the Palm Springs area.

Given this distribution and the modest representation of bisexual women and men and transgender persons, the analyses reported later focus exclusively on gay men and lesbians ($N = 502$). Four age groups were created for analyses: Those younger than 50 years of age (18%; $N = 90$; 69 gay men and 21 lesbians, about one-third of whom in total were younger than 30), those aged 50 to 59 years (26%; $N = 129$; 93 gay men and 36 lesbians), those aged 60 to 69 years (36%; $N = 181$; 148 gay men and 33 lesbians), and those over the age of 70 (20%; $N = 102$; 91 gay men and 11 lesbians, about one-fourth of whom were over the age of 80). A series of

TABLE 1 Demographic Description of Total Sample[a]

Variable	No.	%
Gender/sexual orientation		
Gay male	401	70.5
Lesbian	101	17.7
Bisexual male	14	2.4
Bisexual female	6	1.1
Transgender male-to-female	1	0.2
Straight male	6	1.1
Straight female	40	7.0
Age group		
21–29	6	1.1
30–39	29	5.1
40–49	73	12.8
50–59	139	24.4
60–69	202	35.5
70–79	91	16.0
80–89	27	4.8
90+	2	0.3
Race		
African American	3	0.5
Asian/Pacific Islander	16	2.8
Hispanic/Latino	22	3.9
Native American	7	1.2
Caucasian/White	505	88.8
Other	16	2.8

[a]Numbers based on completed surveys; analytic sample size is a subset.

analyses were conducted using race (dichotomized as Caucasian vs. other) as a variable on all of the dependent variables described later; no significant effects were noted.

Respondents were queried as to their level of fear related to self-identifying as being LGBT (now lesbian or gay, given the groups analyzed). Almost one-third (31.3%) indicated that they had some level of fear (summing the responses of *yes* and *somewhat*) about being open about their sexual orientation. Analyses revealed that fear was not related to age group but was marginally related to gender/sexual orientation, $\chi^2(2, N = 495) = 5.733$, $p = .05$. Lesbians reported that they feared being open about being LGBT more so than did gay men, with respective percentages of 29% and 18.5%. In a follow-up probe, this gender/sexual orientation difference emerged in a stronger way; 66.2% of the lesbians in the sample reported that their fear level varied by context (i.e., the "circumstance or environment" and their "perceived level of acceptance" in that situation) as compared with 52.3% of gay men, $\chi^2(1, N = 405) = 4.752$, $p < .05$. There were no effects attributable to age.

Respondents were next queried about what factors would affect their selection of a community in which to live or visit. Ninety-two percent felt it was somewhat or very important that their sexual orientation/gender identity would be accepted in their chosen community or area, while 6% indicated that it was not a factor in their choice. Consistent with the results reported earlier, analyses indicated that lesbians felt that acceptance in/by their chosen community was more important than did gay men, $\chi^2(2, N = 493) = 11.953$, $p < .005$. Just over 78% of lesbians (78.2%) felt that acceptance was very important, 19.8% felt it was somewhat important, and 2.0% felt it was not important; comparable percentages for gay men were 60.7%, 30.9%, and 8.4%. As mentioned earlier, these results were independent of age.

A similar question asked about the extent to which the respondent's sexual orientation or gender identity would be a factor in their comfortable use of social service targeted to older adults. No significant age or sexual orientation effects were noted. Across gay men and lesbians of all ages, about one-fourth of respondents reported that their sexual orientation would make them uncomfortable accessing the social services targeted to older adults, in general.

A separate, specific question was subsequently posed inquiring if respondents would be more comfortable using social services if an agency providing social services identified as "gay friendly" or "LGBT friendly." Almost 80% (79.1%) indicated that they would feel more comfortable using the services if the service provider was identified in such a way (including the presence of the Rainbow Flag). There was a marginal effect attributable to gender/sexual orientation, $\chi^2(2, N = 483) = 5.729$, $p = .05$: Lesbians were more likely to report that they would be more comfortable using such a social service (74.5%) than were gay men (62.1%). Age group also emerged as a significant effect, $\chi^2(6, N = 437) = 18.849$, $p < .01$. The oldest respondents were less likely than younger respondents to report that they would be more comfortable—that is, among those aged 70 and older, just over one-half (54.5%) reported that they would be more comfortable using the services of an agency identified in such a way; among those in the youngest age group (< 50 years of age), almost three-fourths (74.7%) reported that they would be more comfortable along with 70.7% of those in their 50s and 60.5% of those in their 60s. In contrast, 31.7% of respondents aged 70 and older reported that it would *not* make a difference; again, the comparable percentage for those in youngest age group was 18.1% (with 12.2% and 23.3% the respective percentages for those in their 50s and 60s).

In addition, over 80% (84.2%) indicated that their decision to use services would be possibly or definitely influenced by promotional materials, such as brochures and pamphlets, which included representations of "gay couples." More specific analyses revealed comparable age effects to those reported earlier, $\chi^2(6, N = 430) = 18.651$, $p < .005$—that is, among those aged 70 and older, under one-half (46.9%) reported that they would be more comfortable using the services of an agency that had, in its promotional materials, representations of gay couples; the comparable percentage for those in the youngest age groups was 65.9% (with both other age groups around (63%). In parallel, 21.4% of respondents aged 70 and older reported that it would *not* make a difference; again, the comparable percentages for those in younger age groups ranged from 8.25% (for those younger than 50 years), to 10.7% (for those in their 50s), to 20.1% (for those in their 60s). No gender/sexual orientation differences were noted.

These comfort levels were also associated with the extent to which individuals felt that acceptance in their chosen community was important; treating these measures as continuous, correlations were computed between feeling accepted by one's chosen community and the perceived comfort in using social services, both generally and LGBT-identified. Not surprisingly, those who rated as important the acceptance of one's chosen community were more likely to report that they would feel more comfortable accessing social services identified as LGBT, $r(476) = .383$, $p < .001$; and more likely to have their decision to use social services influenced by the inclusion of LGBT persons in their promotional material, $r(467) = .332$, $p < .001$.

Respondents were also asked if they participated in any LGBT organizations as well as senior social organizations. In response to the focus on LGBT organizations, no significant age group or sexual orientation differences emerged, although, as might be expected, there was a nonsignificant trend ($p = .08$) for the youngest participants (< 50 years of age) to participate *less* often (59.5% reported participating) than those in the older three age groups (for which participation rates were all $> 70\%$). In response to the latter focus on senior social organizations, significant age and sexual orientation differences emerged. Not surprisingly, the oldest participants (i.e., those aged 70 and older) were significantly more likely to participate in senior social organizations (63.5%) than were younger participants (with percentages of 25.3%, 24.2%, and 40.2% for the younger three age groups, respectively); $\chi^2(3, N = 431) = 42.251$, $p < .001$. Gay men were significantly more likely to participate in senior social organizations than were lesbians with respective percentages of 42.1% and 23.2%, $\chi^2(1, N = 470) = 11.550$, $p < .001$.

When asked for additional comments regarding issues, concerns, or services they would like considered in the future planning of the Office on Aging, three general themes emerged, independent of age and sexual orientation:

1. Affordable LGBT affirming elder housing (33%).
   Exemplary quotes that reflect this theme include:
   - "Concerned about LGBT assisted living availability or adult living communities (over 55) and affordable housing for seniors LGBT."
   - "Low income housing in a comprehensive center offering senior center activities and assisted living . . . ."
   - "I see the need for senior gay housing and communities as the baby boomers enter the senior years."

- "Employ LGBT persons on your staff. Make them part of your decision making process. Don't be reluctant to realize that the Coachella Valley is filled with LGBT seniors. Thank you."

2. Recognition and respect of LGBT older persons (28%).
   Exemplary quotes that reflect this theme include:
   - "Gay older adults are subject to being 'invisible' as are all older adults. However, the level or lack of recognition in media, services, etc. is much higher for gay older adults."
   - "A sense of community and camaraderie I think is very important for older LGBT individuals. An organization/setting specifically devoted to older LGBT individuals would meet this need."

3. LGBT-affirmative social services and medical care (26%).
   Exemplary quotes reflecting this theme include:
   - "Assistance as we seniors lose our ability to cope with daily chores, driving socializing, we (some of us) like to be with people like ourselves to talk as we wish rather than skirt around issues."
   - "More organizations for gay women legal aid, more help to make seniors aware of scams, mail fraud, people who prey on older women."
   - "Don't allow social workers to wear or display any religious symbols such as crosses, crucifixes or jewelry that says "Jesus" etc. The County is full of these types of symbols."

DISCUSSION

The foregoing analyses focus on levels of disclosure, comfort, and use of various social service and related settings primarily among LGBT midlife and older adults. Results reveal that older gay men and lesbians maintain some fear of openly disclosing their sexual orientation, although this was not the predominant response and it varied by circumstance and gender. Along comparable lines with similar proportions, older gay men and lesbians maintain some discomfort in their use of older adult social services, even as the majority report that they would feel more comfortable accessing LGBT-friendly identified services and programs; as reported earlier, gender exerted an influence—as did age. The qualitative data aid in the interpretation of these quantitative patterns. These issues, along with actions underway to address their impact, form the focus of the discussion that follows.

Disclosure and Acceptance

The analyses reported earlier reveal the ongoing concerns about disclosure and acceptance. Approximately one-third of these gay and lesbian adults, over 94% of who were at least 40 years of age, reported "some fear" in openly identifying as a gay or lesbian person. Age did not exert an influence on this reported fear, although gender did: Lesbians were more likely to report some fear of disclosure than were gay men. Although not specified, this reported fear varied by the perceived circumstance and environment in which these adults were located; as reported earlier, lesbians were more likely to report such fear than were gay men. This ongoing fear, and the associated sensitivity to the environments and circumstances of interactions, echoes what many authors have noted as the insidious and pervasive influences of minority stress (e.g., Meyer, 2003) and the life-long process of "coming out" (de Vries & Blando, 2004).

Several reports have noted alarmingly high rates of violence and abuse to which LGBT persons are exposed (e.g., Fredriksen-Goldsen et al., 2011; Herek, Gillan, & Cogan, 1999) often noting the culture of discrimination that characterize the lives of (older) LGBT persons and the distal, objective events confronted. The ongoing fears and vigilance reported earlier may be understood in this context as evidence of the proximal, subjective stressors faced by LGBT persons (Meyer, 2003), particularly in the second half of life. That gender may moderate these patterns is intriguing and merits further attention.

Related to this pattern, the vast majority of respondents (92%) reported that feeling accepted is important in the choice of a community to live or to visit. As reported earlier, lesbians more strongly endorsed this view than did gay men. In the context of minority stress and the ongoing effort it takes to be vigilant and to address one's fears of being a sexual minority in a culture that is often unwelcoming, feeling accepted provides respite— the experience of "letting one's guard down." Meyer, Ouellette, Haile, and McFarlane (2011) evocatively studied the responses of 57 sexual minority men and women to this question: "What do you think your life would be like without homophobia, racism, and sexism?" Their responses are relevant here, revealing the many costs of non-acceptance—that is, the respondents commented that homophobia meant that "I could not be myself," as one gay man expressed; and having to "speak in third person invisible," as a lesbian noted. Acceptance reduces these impediments to authenticity; acceptance means not having to worry about the consequences of rejection—of not having to worry about "what's going to happen if somebody knows or finds out" (Meyer et al., 2011, p. 210). Stated as such, it seems reasonable that the majority of midlife and older respondents would note the importance of acceptance in choosing a community.

Acceptance and Social Service Utilization

Two questions were posed addressing the ways in which agencies and social services presented themselves and the perceived level of comfort lesbian and gay midlife and older adults expressed using such agencies and services. Respondents were much more likely (77%) to use social services if the service provider was identified as "gay friendly" or "LGBT friendly." A closely related question inquired if the decision to use such a service or agency would be influenced by the inclusion of images (such as "gay couples"); the results were comparable with almost 85% acknowledging that it would have effect. These data reinforce the importance of acceptance as noted earlier, as well as imply some of the apprehension experienced by LGBT persons in interacting with the social and health service sector, as the free response themes reveal. Clearly, organizations and agencies could benefit from this information as they reach out to a diverse client base, inclusive of LGBT persons.

The understanding of this association, however, is more complex as noted in the additional effects of gender and especially age. Women reported being somewhat more likely to use those services publicly identified as LGBT friendly. This follows on the evocative gender differences in reported acceptance and the likelihood of use of services identified as LGBT noted earlier with little existing research to assist in the interpretation of these effects. Perhaps some of this difference may lie in the setting in which this study was conducted, known to be LGBT-friendly, and disproportionately populated by gay men. Perhaps part of what the midlife and older lesbians are noting through these findings is the desire to be represented not only alongside heterosexual persons, but also alongside gay men.

Age also emerged as a factor in the perceived comfort level and likelihood of service use based on LGBT representation; relative to younger gay men and lesbians, older persons were significantly *less* likely to be drawn to an LGBT designation or by the presentation of "gay couples" on publicity. This speaks to the age-based diversity within even older LGBT populations. Recall that Rawls (2004) found that the proportion of gay men who have disclosed their sexual orientation to many in their environment decreased as a function of age, with older gay men disclosing to fewer than younger gay men. In a related fashion, we (Adelman, Gurevitch, de Vries, & Blando, 2006) have noted this in previous research as well wherein older gay men, for example, were more likely to identify as "homosexual" and less likely to identify as "queer" than were much younger participants. Older lesbians, comparably, were much more likely to identify as "gay" than were younger same gender loving women. Along with degree and frequency, the terms of disclosure differentiate individuals of different ages, different cohorts. The language used, including the images presented, speaks volumes about culture, values, beliefs, and customs and, as such, the extent to which an individual may be welcome and included.

Language and Acknowledgment of LGBT Elders

In response to an open-ended probe addressing other concerns they sought to raise to better prepare for and work with LGBT older persons, respondents echoed many of the issues noted earlier often within the context of respect, and the language and images of inclusion (and exclusion). A prominent theme in the narratives responses was the desire for affordable—and *affirmative*—LGBT senior housing. Housing has become a lightening rod of sorts for LGBT elders (de Vries, 2006), with discussions often contrasting existing heteronormative facilities for older adults with a need for inclusive facilities and services that honor LGBT older adults and diverse life trajectories. The comments by the participants in this study reinforce this point and imply, explicitly in some instances, the need to include LGBT persons as decision-makers and care providers in such settings. Presumably, such inclusion would render a setting more comfortable (as queried in the survey questions reported earlier).

Elaborating on this theme (notwithstanding the age-ambivalent findings around the inclusion of LGBT older adults in promotional materials), respondents also noted the invisibility of LGBT elders in media (and elsewhere); suggestions were offered that a sense of connection could be afforded through organizations and settings that are directly tailored to LGBT older adults (along the lines of SAGE and its many national affiliates). Such settings could afford an authentic pool of support ("We like to be with people like ourselves to talk as we wish rather than skirt around issues," as one respondent noted); such settings could also address the presentation of images that are perceived as exclusionary, as noted in the third theme of the open-ended comments.

The experience of, fears about, and calls for acceptance underlie these patterns and form the key concept of the prior analyses, both qualitative and quantitative. Age and gender/sexual orientation influence these patterns in ways that merit further attention and remind us that "One size does not fit all"; still, the general trend calls for efforts to better reach out to lesbian and gay elders (and LGBT elders more generally).

Limitations and Summary

As with other surveys, there are limitations to the work reported here. Defining a population by sexual orientation or gender identity is complex. Furthermore, there is a great deal of (often unrecognized) diversity within the LGBT elder population regarding culture, ethnicity, education, income, health, and other factors that need to be considered when targeting research and interventions towards these individuals. Moreover, the sample was generated through public venues, precluding access to "harder-to-reach" persons and groups, and favoring those already "out" and availing themselves of LGBT public activities. The questionnaire was brief, designed for easy administration but with associated with costs of data depth. These limitations notwithstanding, the level of fear about being open about one's sexual orientation, concerns about comfortably and authentically accessing care, and desires for LGBT affirmative (at least) services, demand attention.

Faced with widespread homophobia and heterosexism among program staff and heterosexual peers, many LGBT seniors either shun needed services or may not be forthcoming about their sexuality or relationships (Grant, Koskovich, Frazer, & Bjerk, 2009). Heterosexism, or the presumption that all elders are heterosexual, among healthcare providers and social service organizations, can create a norm of "invisibility" for LGBT seniors. In this unwelcoming environment, it is more likely that LGBT seniors will experience barriers to accessing healthcare and social services (Zians, 2004).

Issues facing LGBT seniors are in many ways similar to those of all seniors. Both groups are concerned with maintaining independence, finances, security, social support, health and combating loneliness (MetLife, 2010). In addition to these challenges, however, LGBT seniors are confronted with additional serious barriers to successful aging. These barriers stem from lifetime social stigmatization and discrimination, laws and regulations that contribute to marginalization, and institutionalized homophobia, and transphobia. These experiences of exclusion, in many settings and at multiple levels, have been noted to place LGBT seniors at elevated risk for poverty, homelessness, isolation, and poorer health outcomes than their heterosexual peers (Movement Advancement Project, 2010).

Thus, the need for action on the results of this survey and others more elaborate is acute—that is, insuring a welcoming environment for service access, reducing fear of sexual orientation/gender identity discrimination, and offering culturally competent care is required to address the needs of aging LGBT persons—and a minimum for all agencies seeking to be inclusive and serving a diverse aging population.

ACTIONS UNDERTAKEN AND FUTURE DIRECTIONS

With the passage of AB 2920 Older Californians Equality and Protection Act (2002), and the signature of the governor in 2006, the State of California directed AAA to address the particular needs of senior LGBT persons in their planning and service areas and strategic planning processes. It amended the Welfare and Institutions Code, requiring the California Department of Aging (CDA) to ensure that all programs administered by CDA and the AAA, of which RCOA is one, to address the needs of LGBT elders (AB 2920 Older Californians, 2002). It further directs the CDA to provide technical assistance to the AAA regarding the unique needs of LGBT seniors. The Office on Aging has taken the mandate of AB2920 seriously and has aggressively sought out marginalized LGBT seniors to engage them in the needs assessment and planning process. In addition, the Office on Aging has offered sensitivity training for its staff, Advisory Council, and community and county partners.

In response to this groundbreaking legislation, the RCOA has taken a lead role in meeting the requirements of the law by assessing the current needs of the County's LGBT seniors while concurrently engaging local service providers in a series of trainings on how to better provide for this underserved and understudied population.

There are several areas that would help inform a discussion about needs specific to the LGBT elder community. The first is to support and expand further research into LGBT senior needs. This can be achieved by expanding survey questions and conducting a comprehensive needs assessment of LGBT elders living in Riverside County. Attempts should be made to gather responses from more diverse groups of people including racial minorities, more women as well as bisexual and transgender individuals. Needed in the assessment is a better representation of respondents from other regions of the county. Also, the survey should be expanded to include individuals in their forties to understand their anticipated needs, barriers, and hopes as they will be the next group to utilize social services. A concise evaluation of already existing services and their utilization by LGBT seniors is also needed.

Such a needs assessment can inform the development of curricula to train service providers on the particular needs of the LGBT community including awareness and sensitivity. The assessment can also be used to support civic leaders in the establishment of non-discrimination policies, and to encourage Riverside County agencies, businesses and community based organizations to recognize and support LGBT seniors and their families.

Finally, it is the hope that an LGBT senior planning group will be established to identify and set priorities. This group could work in partnership with the RCOA to conduct periodic needs assessments. In addition, they could provide focus group access and serve as a way to network with community organizations and social services. The dissemination of this report is clearly a place to begin—to assist in framing discussions and charting courses of action and pathways to services and supports for those LGBT elders who are fearful or distrustful of traditional social service delivery systems.

REFERENCES

AB 2920 Older Californians Equality and Protection Act. (2002). *Fact sheet*. San Francisco, CA: Equality California. Retrieved from www.eqca.org

Adelman, M., Gurevitch, J., de Vries, B., & Blando, J. (2006). Openhouse: Community building and research in the LGBT aging population. In D. Kimmel, T. Rose, & S. David (Eds.), *Lesbian, gay, bisexual, and transgender aging: Research and clinical perspectives* (pp. 247–264). New York, NY: Columbia University Press.

Bonvicini, K. A., & Perlin, M. J. (2003). The same but different: Clinician–patient communication with gay and lesbian patients. *Patient Education and Counseling, 51*, 115–122.

Brotman, S., Ryan, B., & Cornier, R. (2003). The health and social service needs of gay and lesbian elders and their families in Canada. *Gerontologist, 43*, 192–202.

Cahill, S., South, K., & Spade, J. (2000). *Outing age: Public policy issues affecting gay, lesbian, bisexual and transgender elders*. Washington, DC: Policy Institute of the National Gay and Lesbian Task Force. Retrieved from www.thetaskforce. org

de Vries, B. (2006). Home at the end of the rainbow: Supportive housing for LGBT elders. *Generations, 29*, 64–69.

de Vries, B., & Blando, J. (2004). The study of gay and lesbian aging: Lessons for social gerontology. In G. Herdt & B. de Vries (Eds.), *Gay and lesbian aging: Research and future directions* (pp. 3–28). New York, NY: Springer.

Fredriksen-Goldsen, K. I., Kim, H.-J., Emlet, C. A., Muraco, A., Erosheva, E. A., Hoy-Ellis, C. P., . . . Petry, H. (2011). *The aging and health report: Disparities and resilience among lesbian, gay, bisexual, and transgender older adults*. Seattle, WA: Institute for Multigenerational Health.

Gates, G. J. (2010). *Sexual minorities in the 2008 general social survey: Coming out and demographic characteristics*. Los Angeles, CA: Williams Institute.

Gates, G. J., & Cooke, A. (2011). *California census snapshot: 2010*. Los Angeles, CA: Williams Institute.

Grant, J., Koskovich, G., Frazer, S., & Bjerk, S. (2009). *Outing Age 2010: Public policy issues affecting lesbian, gay, bisexual and transgender elders*. Washington, DC: National Gay and Lesbian Task Force. Retrieved from www.thetaskforce.org

Herek, G. M., Gillis, J. R., & Cogan, J. C. (1999). Psychological sequelae of hate-crime victimization among lesbian, gay, and bisexual adults. *Journal of Consulting and Clinical Psychology, 67*, 945–951.

Knochel, A., Croghan, C., Moone, R., & Quam, J. (2010). *Ready to serve? The aging network of L, G, B and T older adults*. St. Paul, MN: Author. Retrieved from www.n4a.org/pdf/ReadyToServe1.pdf

Lambda Legal. (2010). *When health care isn't caring: Lambda legal's survey of discrimination against LGBT people and people with HIV*. New York, NY: Author. Retrieved from www.lambdalegal.org/health-care-report

MetLife Mature Market Institute. (2010). *Still out, still aging: The MetLife study of lesbian, gay, bisexual and transgender baby boomers*. Westport, CT: Author.

Meyer, I. H. (2003). Prejudice, social stress, and mental health in lesbian, gay, and bisexual populations: Conceptual issues and research evidence. *Psychological Bulletin, 129*, 674–697.

Meyer, I. H., Ouellette, S. C., Haile, R., & McFarlane, T. A. (2011). "We'd be free": Narratives of life without homophobia, racism, or sexism. *Sexuality Research and Social Policy, 8*, 204–214.

Movement Advancement Project. (2010). *Improving the lives of LGBT older adults*. New York, NY: SAGE and the Movement Advancement Project.

National Resource Center on LGBT Aging. (2010). *LGBT older adults and exclusion from aging services and programs*. New York, NY: Sage. Retrieved from http://www.lgbtagingcenter.org/resources/pdfs/LGBTOlderAdultsandExclusionfrom AgingPrograms.pdf

Rawls, T. (2004). Disclosure and depression among older gay and homosexual men: Findings from the Urban Men's Health Study. In G. Herdt & B. de Vries (Eds.), *Gay and lesbian aging: Research and future directions* (pp. 117–142). New York, NY: Springer.

Romero, A. P., Rosky, C. J., Badgett, M. V., Lee, M. V., & Gates, G. J. (2008). *Census snapshot: California*. Los Angeles, CA: Williams Institute. Retrieved from http://escholarship.org/uc/item/4xq120m0

Zians, J (2004). *The San Diego County LGBT senior healthcare needs assessment*. San Diego, CA: Alliance Healthcare Foundation. Retrieved from http://www.sage-sd.com/SeniorNeedsAssessment

Aging Out: A Qualitative Exploration of Ageism and Heterosexism Among Aging African American Lesbians and Gay Men

IMANI WOODY, PhD

Mary's House for Older Adults, Inc., Washington, DC, USA

African Americans elders, like their non-African American counterparts, are not a homogeneous group; however an early characteristic placed on all African Americans is in their shared history in the United States. As members of multiple minority groups, older lesbian, gay, bisexual, and transgender (LGBT) people of African descent have survived racism, heterosexism, homophobia, and now ageism. This article describes a qualitative study grounded in Black feminist and minority stress theories that explored the issues of perceived social discrimination and alienation of 15 older African American lesbians and gay males whose lived experiences were captured using in-depth, face-to-face interviews. Several themes were identified in the study, including (a) Sense of Alienation in the African American Community, (b) Deliberate Concealment of Sexual Identity and Orientation, (c) Aversion to LGBT Labels, (d) Perceived Discrimination and Alienation From Organized Religion, (e) Feelings of Grief and Loss Related to Aging, (f) Isolation, and (g) Fear of Financial and Physical Dependence. The implication of the findings suggests that the ethos and needs of older African American lesbian women and gay men need to be addressed to eliminate potential barriers to successful aging for this cohort.

Despite impressive advances on many fronts, the systematic injustices based on one's race, gender identity, sexual orientation and age remain. These injustices can create an at-risk environment for older lesbian, gay, bisexual, and transgender (LGBT) African Americans, widening the gap of disparities in economics, health care, employment, housing, education, and their over-all quality of life. Evidence shows that many African Americans growing up before, during and after the Civil Rights Movement experienced bla-tant, overt racism (Smith, 2007). Similarly, LGBT older people have lived through criminalization and psychiatric diagnosis of their sexual identity and sexual orientation culminating in lost jobs, housing, children and even their lives. In addition, older persons, and perhaps especially LGBT older people, have endured the stigma, prejudice, and discrimination related to aging in a youth oriented society. As a consequence of this perceived and actual racism, homophobia, heterosexism, and ageism, many LGBT African Americans are reticent and are unable to access sensitive and appropriate services to support themselves and their families (González, 2007).

This article reports on a qualitative exploration ($n = 15$) using Giorgi's (1997) empirical Phenomenological Model to explore the psychosocial issues and needs that can accompany aging as a Black[1], lesbian or gay male; this includes the possible challenges that can arise for this group when accessing social and community-based services (including religious institutions). The findings suggest that the ethos of older African American lesbian women and gay men should be addressed to eliminate potential barriers to suc-cessful aging in and access to community-based settings including long-term care facilities, health and treatment centers, and spiritual and recreational spaces. Recommendations to achieve parity in access to services and the development of a genuine welcoming environment are presented.

LITERATURE REVIEW

Much of the research conducted for lesbian women and gay men has been described as centered on the experiences of White, formally educated, mid-dle class lesbian and gay individuals (Gabbay & Wahler, 2002; Szymanski & Gupta, 2009; Woolf, 1998). There is a scarcity of empirical investiga-tions that examine the intersection of aging, sexual orientation and gender identity among Black lesbian women and gay men. Currently, 12.6% of the United States population is African American (U.S. Census Bureau, 2012) with expectations of comparable proportions among LGBT persons (although this remains an empirical question); however representation of older African American lesbian women and gay men are nearly imperceptible (Fish, 2007).

African Americans as a group experience major gaps in health and financial security (American Association of Retired Persons, 2010). African American elders are most likely to experience poverty, with poverty rates more than twice that of all other older Americans (Beedon & Wu, 2004). There is now a sizable literature documenting the systematic discrimination experienced by African Americans (Azibo, 1989; Collins, 2000, Neville, Coleman, Falconer, & Holmes, 2005); analyses have suggested that exposure to such discrimination, including media portrayals of negative aging stereotypes, is associated with negative health conditions (Levy, 2005, as cited in Currey, 2008). These conditions may be exacerbated in the lives of older Black LGBT persons, however, in their either misrepresentation or, more commonly, under-representation in media and related images of all sorts. The messages of these infrequent or skewed images fuel misconceptions, hostilities, shame, and non-acceptance in the social scripts and societal norms of the United States (National Gay and Lesbian Task Force, 2009).

Of particular concern is research by Szymanski and Gupta (2009) that revealed African American lesbians and gay males experience multiple minority stressors through their exposure to multiple forms of oppression, both from mainstream "White" culture and the African American heterosexual community. Wilson and Miller (2002) stated it this way:

> Members of ethnic minority groups must develop unique cognitive and behavioral strategies to manage stress, cope with institutionalized and overt racism, and mitigate the negative psychological outcomes that result from living in an oppressive environment. Particular minority groups such as African American bisexual and gay men must learn to cope with two distinct forms of oppression: heterosexism and racism. (p. 371)

Other research found that African values of spirituality, collectivity, sharing, and a reverence for older adults permeates African American culture and recognized that the role of older African Americans includes the modeling of attitudes and behaviors deemed appropriate (Strom, Carter, & Schmidt, 2004). In fact, research indicates that a majority of African Americans are closely connected psychologically and culturally with their racial and ethnic communities from birth and are supported as members of these communities. However, sexual identity and sexual orientation are not similarly supported (Szymanski & Gupta, 2009).

Accordingly, the risk of losing one's support from the African American racial and ethnic communities because of perceived homosexual or bisexual and questioning identity and orientation can be devastating with significant social and health implications (Wilson & Miller, 2002). Aging LGBT African Americans face unique challenges regarding discrimination and access to social and community-based services, access to health care, housing, community resources, and familial, financial and legal supports and security (Grant, 2010). This study examines these particular issues among aging African American lesbian woman and gay men through the lived experiences of representatives of this cohort.

METHOD

A qualitative, phenomenological design was engaged to explore the psychosocial issues of aging of 15 older African American lesbians and gay males through their lived experiences (Giorgi, 1997). By using this model, the study intended to capture the voices of a marginalized group that is generally missing from research (Grant, 2010). It specifically permitted an analysis of the intersections of age, race, and sexual orientation on their effects on accessing community-based programs.

Prior to and during the data collection, the researcher adopted the phenomenological "attitude of reduction" or epoche process that required her to bracket any preconceived notions, thoughts, or biases in collecting and analyzing the data (Kostere, Kostere, & Percy, 2009). While the researcher served as the primary tool, the in-depth personal interview was guided by a series of open-ended questions allowing the creation of Level I[2] in the Giorgi (1997) empirical Phenomenological Model.

This modality is often used in community-based needs assessments and was chosen to capture more fully the lived experiences of this cohort. The instrument included queries that sought to initiate discussions on daily and eventual social supports; determine (if there were) potential barriers to accessing community services and supports because of age, sexual identity, or sexual orientation; and record their lived experiences navigating through society as old, lesbian, and gay male African Americans. It was reviewed by panel of experts in the field of lesbian women and gay male issues.

Description of Sample and Recruitment

Using purposive sampling, 11 females and 4 males of African descent, ranging in ages from 58 to 72 years of age were recruited from two purposefully selected sites: a national health organization and a midsized, Christian-based church. Both entities provide or assist in providing community-based social services and serve many individuals who are African American, identify as a lesbian woman or gay male, and are within the age criteria. In addition, the organization has local programs designed to serve African Americans and elders and the church is beginning an older adults' ministry. The researcher was acquainted with the leaders and contacted the gatekeepers (Creswell, 2007) to explain the nature and scope of the research, including the process and ethical consideration of their members. Both the organization and the church were eager to support the research to further identify the needs of African American elder clients and congregants, respectively, and to ensure an expansive and inclusive outreach to those inside and outside of their physical boundaries.

Each site received and placed institutional review board-approved information about this study in their newsletters and on their Web sites. Moreover, each leader agreed to provide a private space to conduct interviews and to identify other venues to announce the opportunity to participate in the study. Respondents were contacted by the researcher via e-mail or by telephone to complete the initial interview screening. Upon meeting the criteria the participants were given the option to meet at a site of their choice.

Of the 15 people of African descent in the sample, four identified their race and ethnicity as Black and eight identified their heritage as African American. One participant identified as a person of Caribbean African American ancestry, another participant identified as biracial (i.e., Caucasian and African American heritage), and one participant identified her ancestry as multiracial (i.e., Native American, Black American, and Caucasian). The median age of the participants was 64 years old and they identified their current socioeconomic status as middle class. Twelve participants were retired, one was semi-retired, and two worked full time.

The sample was highly educated: two participants had doctoral degrees, six participants had master's degrees (one participant had two master's degrees), and seven participants had received advanced technical training or had some college beyond high school. The participants' religious affiliations included Baptist, Unitarian, and Pentecostal, with more than one-half considering themselves Christian. Thirteen participants stated they had relinquished traditional religion and focused on being spiritual and having a personal connection with God. Table 1 provides a fuller description of the sample.

TABLE 1 Participant Code and Demographics

Participant Code	Age	Birth Gender	Employment Status	Education	Socioeconomic Strata	Race Ethnicity
Participant 1	58	Female	Employed	Postgraduate	Middle class	African American
Participant 2	65	Female	Retired	Postgraduate	Middle class	Biracial
Participant 3	69	Male	Semi-retired	PhD	Middle class	Caribbean African American
Participant 4	60	Female	Employed	Postgraduate	Middle class	Black
Participant 5	58	Male	Retired	Some college	Middle class	Black
Participant 6	67	Female	Retired	Some college	Middle class	Multiracial
Participant 7	72	Female	Retired	Some college	Middle class	African American
Participant 8	66	Female	Retired	Some college	Middle class	African American
Participant 9	64	Male	Retired	Postgraduate	Middle class	African American
Participant 10	63	Female	Retired	Some college	Middle class	African American
Participant 11	59	Female	Retired	Some college	Middle class	Black
Participant 12	66	Female	Retired	Some college	Middle class	African American
Participant 13	67	Female	Retired	PhD	Middle class	African American
Participant 14	63	Male	Retired	BA	Middle class	African American
Participant 15	64	Female	Employed	Postgraduate	Middle class	Black

The participants spoke frankly and openly about topics and experiences that were at times very personal and very painful disclosures. All of the participants were enthusiastic about their participation in the study and the possible positive effects of the research on the issues discussed during the interview. The interviews averaged 2 hr in length, and all were audio-recorded and transcribed for the purposes of data analysis.

To minimize bias, the researcher triangulated the data (Creswell, 2007) by using observations, field notes, and the taped interviews. This process produced rich details of the lived experiences of the participants, allowing the researcher to conduct a contemplative analysis and interpretation of the data (Kostere et al., 2009). The data were coded (described later) and cross-referenced. Qualitative software that included data integrity checks was used to provide additional analysis to assure the accuracy and reliability of the sub-themes.

Data Analysis

Giorgi's (1997) Phenomenological Model of analysis required the researcher to use the following five steps when analyzing the data: (a) constructing a sense of the whole, (b) discriminating meaning units within a psychological perspective to focus on the phenomenon being researched, (c) transformating participants' everyday expressions into psychological language with emphasis on the phenomenon being investigated, (d) conducting a synthesis of transformed meaning units into a consistent statement of the structure of the experience, and (e) engaging in a final synthesis (Kostere et al., 2009). The initial coding recognized 54 nodes or meaning units. These nodes were synthesized from the communication nuances of the participants to a more psychological scientific language, thereby completing Level II[3] of the empirical Phenomenological Model (Giorgi, 1997). By applying thematic analysis, the researcher utilized a methodical approach that allowed the findings to become more defined (Kostere et al., 2009). Similar nodes were merged; redundant themes, ideas, and concepts were eliminated. The nodes were then grouped into smaller clusters called themes. Some of the themes identified were classified as outliers because they were not identified by a majority of the participants or were outside of the scope of this research.

RESULTS

Several major themes were identified during this process. They are listed here in the descending order of prevalence: (a) Sense of Alienation in the African American Community, (b) Deliberate Concealment of Sexual Identity and Orientation, (c) Aversion to LGBT Labels, (d) Perceived Discrimination and Alienation From Organized Religion, (e) Feelings of Grief and Loss Related to Aging, (f) Isolation, and (g) Fear of Financial and Physical Dependence.

Sense of Alienation in the African American Community

All of the participants experienced a sense of alienation in the African American community. It was described consistently as "a hurt that lasts a long time." Many experienced this alienation as adolescents because of their budding sexual orientation, perceived identity, or mixed heritage. Participant 14 (male, aged 63) described how his mother received him after being raised by his aunts when he was 13 years old:

> I grew up in North Carolina and moved to Washington when I was 13 . . . . And that was a whole cultural adjustment for me because my mother was expecting this little boy who played baseball and knew how to fix cars and so forth and what she got was a queen who knew Shakespeare and theatre and could sew a button . . . and cook better than she could . . . . So I had to try to fit into her concept of what a little boy should be . . . . And my mother was homophobic big time.

Participant 13 (female, age 67) observed the following about her sexual orientation:

> As I was growing up, I knew enough that you shouldn't speak of it, even if you thought it you don't speak of it. And you assimilate as much as you can. And assimilation meant that you made sure your behavior was above suspicion.

Still others felt this sense of alienation because of the expectations of the community. Participant 5 (male, age 58) elaborated further:

> Well it hurts of course, but again being African American you hurt on two levels at the same time. You hurt because you are Black and you hurt, sometimes you hurt because you are black and gay; you can't separate the two. So you feel hurt, then for me the fear comes in because I [am] again looking like I did when I was younger being attacked and beaten up. I've had things thrown at me as recently as five years ago on the Metro, bottles and stuff. So fear jumps in next because I don't know whether somebody is going to hurt me.

Participant 14 (male, age 63) described feelings of being different because he had a less "manly," more androgynous look:

> One of my issues being African American and looking like this was really when I came out in college in the late 60's at the height of the Black Power Movement and I was distinctly told by a couple of Black organizations at the time we don't want your kind here. So that is one of the most blatant ones [examples of discrimination], we don't want your kind here and I knew exactly what they meant.

All of the participants talked about being conflicted in telling their family members their sexual orientation and sexual identity fearing rejection and abandonment. So it is not surprising that a majority of the participants told their families well into their adult years—after they were 35 years old. Participant 4 (female, age 60) told her parents at age 39:

> I knew I was going to tell my parents, my father was the first one [I came out to]. I thought I'd have more problems with him but it turned out that my mother was ballistic. She didn't want to hear nothing. I was trying to tell her and she just didn't want to hear it. [She] didn't want to get it "I don't wanna hear it." So she played that game; but I didn't back down.

She spoke about an experience with her wife's family:

> They didn't even want to stay in our house when we had a big Thanksgiving celebration because they had two young daughters and I guess they thought we were going to jump them. That's all I can figure.

Six participants experienced overt negative behavior in the African American community and more than one-half had been called names, whispered about or harassed because of being perceived as a gay male or lesbian woman. Participant 5 (male, age 58) shared his experience:

> . . . I was called a faggot on my job. I didn't know about the rights I had back then. That was in my early 20's. Every now and then having a neighbor call me a fag or in the store of something like that but that's about it. Wait a minute, in high school, someone with a big marker put my name up on the wall on the staircase. It said "_____ is gay." Of course I got in the classroom, I stayed there for a little while, I had to go to the bathroom, and I wiped it down. So it was known throughout the school . . . . I have been called faggot on the bus, I have had people . . . I had one guy just get up and move because he thought I was too gay.

These communications from the participants describe deep feelings of alienation from the African American community, which were pervasive and included all levels, from nuclear and extended family, school attendance, church participation, employment, and social endeavors. These experiences of disaffection by the participants often produced estrangement and feelings of fear, sadness and despondency.

Deliberate Concealment of Sexual Identity and Orientation

Only a few of the participants were out to everyone. Fear of rejection and abandonment, or worse, led the remaining participants to state that they did not feel a need to come out to everyone. As a result, they were out to a select number of people who included very close friends and close family members. They were out to others only on a need-to-know basis.

Participants selectively shared sexual status with health professionals. Participant 10 (female, 63), stated it this way: ". . . I don't think my pulmonologist needs to know that I am queer to deal with my lungs . . . ." Participant 12 (female, age 66) communicated her feelings as follows:

> I don't just go into it. If it comes up [I'll share]. I'm African American; you can see that, and a woman. But somehow things happen that comes up and I just say I'm a lesbian . . . . I don't care what they say first do no harm and you're a human being first with biases . . . and who knows . . . once they find out they gonna kill me anyway. Right, so it's a double question mark [gay and Black].

Participant 14 (male, 63), stated it this way:

> You have to be careful because the minute you tell a medical person you are gay, they automatically in 90% of the cases will assume you are HIV positive and start to react that way. And I have had to remind a doctor or two, I'm not positive, I'm negative. I'm gay but I'm negative. So let's stop that train of thought right now!

This deliberate concealment of one's sexual identity and orientation was also present in professionals working with LGBT clients. For example, Participant 15 (female, age 64), a professional counselor, asserted:

> I'm a counselor so I'm not going to have pictures of my family around because people . . . talk about your family . . . and ask you some personal questions that are not necessary. But if I have someone who is gay or lesbian and has some issues of discrimination, I *may* come out to them.

All the participants alluded to the risk it takes to "come out." Many participants perceived that this selective showing of oneself is "the way it is" in the African American community, especially for older people. Many mentioned the strength that is required to make the decision to come out is based on whether they would be treated with respect and dignity and if they perceived calamitous consequences as a result. This thought process seems to be applied to institutions as well as individuals.

Aversion to LGBT Labels

In response to a hostile environment, and consistent with other research (Fish, 2007), many of the African American lesbian women and gay men in this study reported a dislike of the terms lesbian or gay and prefer the terms women who have sex with women; men who have sex with men or same-gender loving. Part of this aversion seems to stem from their experiences of being a recipient of negative usages or seeing others bullied and attacked with these words.

In the study, four females chose the identifier "woman who loves women," one female and one male chose "same gender loving" as descriptors of their sexual orientation. Participant 8 (female, age 66) shared:

> When I was coming up the word was bull dagger. It was so negative . . . I hate that word . . . I just ugh . . . . That's so derogatory. It's negative . . . . [The word] lesbian wasn't there. Gay wasn't there at that time. Those words came later. It was either butch or bull dagger. Most of the time White folks were bull dagger.

Participant 2 (female, age 65) concurs. She stated, "You know I am just a woman that likes feminine women . . . . I am very assertive and don't place myself in any category whatsoever. I don't like dyke; I don't like butch and those are very negative." Participant 11 (female, age 59) responded positively to same-gender loving: "I like that; its [sexual orientation] is not general knowledge." Participant 3 (male, age 69) presented a clear preference for using the words "same-gender-loving":

> I [am] in a same-gender-loving relationship. In other words, I have been in relationships with women and don't rule out the possibility it could happen again. But currently, and [I] have been for a long time, 32 years in a same-gender-loving relationship.

Another participant (male, age 58) labeled himself "macho" and "not flamboyant." Similarly, many participants specifically refused to accept words such as "queer," "butch," "femme," "queen," "lipstick lesbian," "daddy," or "bear" as identifiers. Some participants remarked that their preference for words may be generational as they have heard younger LGBT African Americans refer to themselves as "queer," for example.

Perceived Discrimination and Alienation From Organized Religion

Historically, religion has given this population hope and peace and is an integral part in the lives of African Americans (Fisher, 2007). Accordingly, 14 of the participants considered themselves solely from a Christian background; one participant reported that she was allowed to experiment with different theologies during childhood. Fourteen of the participants engaged in organized religion; all reported such participation provided them some support. Each participant had developed a sense of a benevolent God in their own image. Two participants have become ministers in the New Thought Spiritual Movement and 12 participants embraced a broader sense of spirituality rather than traditional religious teachings.

At the same time, all of the participants voiced frustration at the way the Bible was interpreted to make them feel disenfranchised and without redemption by some church leaders and others. All of the participants had experienced discrimination from organized religion. Four participants felt a sense of alienation from organized religion. Eleven of the participants had experienced discrimination growing up in the church, others experienced it as young adults, and a few continued to experience it in the churches they currently attend. Participant 13 (female, age 67) stated:

> When I was younger, I was raised in the Baptist church and in the Baptist church you were going to hell every Sunday. So there was absolutely no place in your thinking for being anything other than heterosexual.

Participant 7's (female, 72) story echoed the experiences of many in this cohort, of what could and did happen:

> I grew up in the Church. I was baptized when I was about 11 . . . . I came to DC and joined a world-renowned Baptist church. I sang on two choirs, was a part of the missionary group . . . . I met a very nice young lady and we were going to get married so we sent some invitations to people at the church . . . . There were some people on the Deacon and Trustee Board who brought me before the church . . . . We got into this thing about what the Bible did and didn't say, but they put me out anyway . . . . It still hurt me deeply. It was one of the deepest hurts I have had in my life to be put out of my church that I have put so much love and energy . . . .

The majority (12) of participants embraced a broader sense of spirituality rather than traditional religious teachings, often explicitly associated with these experiences of discrimination and alienation. All of the participants used religion or spirituality as a cornerstone of their lives and commented on its importance in providing hope, comfort and peace. Ambivalence may best characterize the relation between organized religion and religious beliefs for this sample.

Feelings of Grief and Loss Related to Aging

Some of the participants expressed sadness as they talked about becoming an old person. Several reported experiencing sadness because of their perception of a lack of reverence for older people and the perception that older people are insignificant in this country. Participant 13 (female, age 67) echoed this sentiment:

> . . . [G]etting old in this country is difficult because we have no reverence for the elderly . . . . So when you add . . . stigma to it now, not only am

I old, I'm an old African American female, and females in this country, at least in my experience has been that you don't enjoy the same reverence as males do and then when you add being a lesbian to that, that puts you already down pretty far, and then when you add being a lesbian to that, that puts you in the toilet.

One person stated he felt like part of a "throw-away society."

Many communicated a sense of grief by not feeling relevant in the mainstream communities and feeling less important in the smaller arenas where they have built relationships. Participant 6 (female, age 67) elaborated:

What I find is like being placated because you are older. I have to say things two and three times, not because they don't hear me, but because they don't see me. It's like I've become invisible or something. When I was younger like even 10 . . . years ago, I would say what I needed to say and people would hear me. And now I have to raise myself and my voice to be heard [she sits straight in her chair to demonstrate] . . . . Because they see my gray hair or see me walking slowly . . . it's like I don't know anything.

Others reported a frustration at having to address still another "ism" (ageism) within their family, work, church, and health care relations. Participant 2 (female, age 65) shared:

They [my cousins] think that physically that I am not able to do things that I used to be able to do and it is very frustrating. Like I reached down to pick up a 4 pound bag and somebody said don't pick that up we don't want you to hurt yourself or . . . teasing me when I want to drive . . . . They don't listen . . . they hear you but they don't listen.

Other participants expressed a loss in terms of health insurance options and the access to services compared to services when they were employed with better insurance options. All of the participants expressed a sense of mortality that assumed center stage as they aged.

For example, one participant stated she didn't think about death and dying when she was younger, but she thinks about it now. She thinks about her death and the death of other people. She stated the death of her close cousin had "such a hard impact" on her own life. She couldn't believe that someone she grew up with and was her age could die. Participant 14 (male, age 63) concurred:

Here's the really hard part for me. Between 1990 and 2000, I lost 100 friends to HIV. My entire social circle are [populated with] people I would have grown old with and be socializing with now are dead. I stopped counting after [the year] 2000. I stopped checking the obits because it just got too overwhelming. My best buddy that I actually hung out with . . . and who came out to me after being married for 10 or 15 years, he died of a heart attack, not HIV [participant begins to cry]. I have three other friends who died of heart attacks again who I would have grown old with. And I have [endured] three suicides.

Whether making reference to their own aging or the aging and the losses of others, the participants in this study adopted a frame of sadness and grief. Some of this has to do with how they are perceived; some of this has to do with how their lives and networks have changed.

Isolation

Several participants experienced isolation from the majority population, variously defined, because of a fear of reprisal, job loss (e.g., dishonorable discharge from military), or disparate treatment. Sometimes the color of one's skin can lead to isolation, even in the LGBT community. Participant 3 (male, age 69) described his experiences:

What happens sometimes is again a feeling of isolation and loneliness of . . . clearly being the only Black sometimes in a group is not always comfortable. For example, I've been going to ____ meetings and sometimes I'm the only Black person there. It just feels weird because whenever they want diversity, it's me, or they expect me to identify some others for them . . . . I[am] . . . a token Black person. [However] . . . we can make it known, "No, I don't want to play that role." That's what I do. And sometimes I do play that role, but I let them know that that's what [I'm doing]. I say, "Oh so this is what you want me to do?" . . . If I think it's important enough to play that role I'll do it, but I'm being very clear that that's what I'm doing.

Here, the isolation is paradoxically in the presence of many others and points to the role and (sometimes absent) experience of authentic inclusion.

Five participants reported self-imposed isolation related to aging that included an unwillingness or inability to drive, limited transportation options, lack of events for their peer group, the lack of compatriots, and chronic ailments and disabilities. Participant 7 (female, age 67) shared the following experience:

I started forgetting things, like people's names and events . . . . My memory changed and arthritis began taking place. I'm doing less than I ever did. I have always been very active, not just sports wise, but as far as doing for other people and doing for myself [participant shakes her head from left to right, while holding her head down]. [Because of] the memory lapses and stuff like that, I don't feel comfortable around people because it takes me so long to think of what I want to say. I can't think of what I want to say; it will come five minutes later. So I don't feel comfortable being in crowds for that reason.

A majority of the participants remarked that they no longer go to clubs or other social venues because of the youth oriented culture, "stares, and unkind comments," the perception of being the oldest person in the room, or finding oneself surrounded by people with whom they had nothing in common. Participant 2 (female, age 65) articulated it this way:

> It's kind of different relating to the younger generation on a social level . . . . They don't even know the music that you prefer, you know and I noticed that. When they were playing the old music, most of them were back there laughing and talking "I wish they would play something else."

As mentioned earlier, isolation derives from several sources and directions, some self-imposed, most other-imposed. The effects are comparable, nonetheless, and are clearly related to the sadness and grief previously described.

Fear of Financial and Physical Dependence

All of the participants expressed a deep anxiety and fear of becoming physically or financially dependent in their later years. Participant 12 (female, age 66) stated:

> My fear is that I won't have the energy to coordinate Meals on Wheels or transportation to and from the hospital. That's [my] great big fear of just being infirmed.

All of the participants feared becoming a burden to others because of physical limitations. Participant 11 (female, age 59) shared:

> My fear is about . . . my independence. My fears [are] not being able to drive, not being able to poop, or urinate, eyesight failing, muscles failing—geeze, medical deterioration. Well my brother already told me if something happens where I can't take care of myself that he would come put me in a nursing home . . . . So my other brother, B. said that he would try to keep me here but I realize that he has his own family . . . and he has a life.

Several participants spoke of not having children or a group of people one can rely on if one became physically or financially dependent. Participant 14 (male, age 63) declared:

> I don't have any family left; all of my family is deceased . . . . So being cared for by others is a fear . . . . So here you are again, at the mercy of someone else who is not a friend.

Many cited seeing the maltreatment of elders as part of the fear of being physically dependent; and some knew of instances wherein LGBT people were treated horribly. Participant 6 (female, age 67) shared of her knowledge of discrimination of LGBT people being cared for in institutions:

> I am a nurse. I really don't want to be incapacitated to the extent that I have to go into one of these facilities because I know first-hand how mean and ugly people can be towards our [LGBT] people . . . . I know a prime example . . . . [He was] physically raped . . . . A lot of people feel that if I complain I still have to live there. There is no telling what else they might do to me . . . .

Equally distressing to this group was a fear of not having enough money to last throughout their lives and the very real possibility of not having good health care and medical services. Participant 12 (female, age 66) said, "My fears are financial [too] and not having money!"

Participant 10 (female, 63) elaborated:

> I don't have any of those things in place in terms of insurance for long-term care [or] insurance for assisted living . . . . This illness is really going to break me. I am probably going to have to dip into any little bit of savings I was trying to accumulate for later on, in order to deal with the medical stuff . . . .

All of the participants hoped they would keep their physical and financial health as they aged because the alternatives were distressing.

DISCUSSION

The vividness and clarity portrayed by the responses of the participants who are also members of the aging population, the African American community and the LGBT community confirm that each is a "knower" of those communities (Grasswick, 2006) and "know" the experiences of isolation, alienation, grief and "otherness." These significant findings are further supported by Black feminist theory whereby the experiences of interlocking oppressions (e.g., racism, ageism, and heterosexism) are considered legitimate and offer additional ways of having knowledge from "outsider-within" positions (Collins, 2000). Indeed, many older lesbian and gay males African Americans must navigate multiple hostile terrains throughout their lives.

These unwelcoming environments can create and perpetuate the development of semi-secret or secret lives and can lead to isolation (Cahill, South, & Spade, 2000).

The participants of this study revealed that throughout their lives they have endured a pervasive sense of "otherness." All of the participants had experienced bigotry based on race and ethnicity and many had experienced and feared discrimination based on sexual orientation and identity as adolescents and adults. Many described feeling depressed because of the reception of the African American community to their lesbian or gay male orientation and identity and the reception of the dominant LGBT community to their racial identity. Many went through "cycles" of internalized homophobia, feeling that being a lesbian or gay male was unfitting and wrong; several report that they could "hide" their sexual orientation but not their racial identity.

Many of the participants experienced being alone and considered themselves as loners early in their lives because of their feeling or sense of being "other." Several participants experienced isolation from the majority population because of a fear of reprisal, job loss (e.g., dishonorable discharge from military), or disparate treatment. Similarly, participants experienced isolation in the LGBT community because they appeared to be older. Two experienced this isolation by often being the only people of color (specifically, African Americans) in LGBT community focused meetings, suggesting that the lack of a people of color involvement was because of the perception that the organization was a "White male" organization. This was confirmed as some lesbian women reportedly found many events were "too male and too White."

Participants also reported self-imposed isolation related to aging that included an unwillingness or inability to drive, limited transportation options, chronic ailments and disabilities, lack of events for their peer group, the lack of compatriots, and a youth-oriented culture. All conveyed an uneasiness of growing older in a perceived hostile environment. More than one-half of the participants remarked that they no longer go to clubs or other social venues because of the "stares, and unkind comments," the perception of being the oldest person in the room, or finding oneself surrounded by people with whom she or he had nothing in common. Interesting to note however, is that a majority of the participants perceived racism as a constant in their lives and more insidious than ageism or heterosexism. Their lack of acceptance by and connection to multiple communities jeopardize their wellbeing and sense of self.

Implications

Amid this "otherness" and its many costs, it is important to understand that older African American lesbian and gay males as a group also present great resilience. Many have lived through Jim Crow and the Civil Rights era. All have developed strategies to live less encumbered lives. Several in this study remarked on how getting older freed them up to say no (or yes) and to do some things that they had been hesitant to do in their youth. Many agreed that challenges based on racial or gender oppression made it easier to deal with oppression based on age. Many have a highly developed network of people whom they call family of choice or what the author terms as logical family. This cohort also has a history of "feeling other" and in response has developed a keen sense of who (individuals) and what (organizations) are inclusive and welcoming. Many developed this sagacity by experiencing hostile environments as children and young adults.

It should be recognized that older African American lesbian women and gay men can face constant stigma and systemic bigotry that in turn can create challenges for integration of their lesbian, gay, and aging selves into society. It is important for those who work with or serve this population to consider that many members of this cohort have experienced injurious events and rejection (Kertzner, Meyer, Frost, & Stirratt, 2009; Moradi et al., 2010) and may find it difficult to access social and community-based services. Barriers to participation in mainstream environments included assumed heterosexuality, lack of respect for one's personhood, fear of being harassed or discriminated by the staff or others, fear of being outed, and the lack of LGBT and African American cultural sensitivity markers in the physical environment (Pope, Wierzalis, Barrett, & Rankin, 2007).

This study found that in African American communities, the most common indicator to ascertain the LGBT and aging friendliness of organizations (including churches) is word of mouth corroboration and the organization's external markers of inclusivity. (This study also validated that this process is used to determine racial and ethnic receptiveness.) Those markers could include positive messaging of age, race, and sexual orientation in mission statements, advertisements, staff attitudes and the physical environment. Therefore agencies should actively acknowledge, accept, and welcome the presence of older African American lesbian women and gay men through all of their communications. Such communications should be built on knowledge that has been acquired in this and other research and not assumptions. Training of organizational staff using culturally competent curriculum that specifically addresses the needs of aging LGBT elders including the nuances within the aging African American LGBT is recommended.

It was interesting to note that the participants considered their racial identity to be more important than their other identities including gender and sexual identity/orientation. This was illustrated repeatedly when the participants talked about their place in African American society and the larger culture. For that reason, it is important that programs that serve older persons, African Americans and LGBT individuals acknowledge and affirm the lived experiences of this population especially as they offer a respite from loneliness, depression and internalized homophobia. In addition, an organization or agency would increase its credibility and viability to this group by becoming aware of and involved with issues important to them such as an increase of HIV/AIDS cases among African Americans and supportive allies to end economic, financial, health, and education disparities; and all-inclusive practices and procedures should include a sincere respect for differences and ongoing cultural sensitive awareness training based on race, gender identity, and sexual orientation.

Limitations

This study is limited by its small sample size and the composition of the participants. Indeed, all of the participants in this study self-identified as middle class, and a majority reported fairly high levels of education. Their middle class status and advanced education may have buffered the participants, to some degree, from the environments of assumed heterosexuality and ageism. However, the makeup of the participants in this study resemble other studies that used "volunteer-based samples of LGBQ [lesbian, gay, bisexual, and queer] persons and consistent with studies that lesbians and gay men, on average are better educated than their heterosexual counterparts" (Szymanski & Gupta, 2009, p. 116).

Moreover, all the participants lived in the metropolitan Washington, DC area and their experiences reflect those of persons living in a more urban setting. This environment is often more accepting of lesbian women and gay men and has more LGBT African American specific organizations in which to buffer prejudicial and discriminatory behavior than small towns and rural settings. Another limitation was the documented reluctance of this cohort to identify as lesbian and gay male and to admit to being 55 years of age or older (Woody, 2008). As a result, only one participant in this study was older than 70 years.

A potential limitation could have been the researcher's self-disclosure as a lesbian woman to the participants. This disclosure could have created the possibility of a contamination of the participants' responses in an effort to please the researcher. However, such biases were addressed by a triangulation of the data. Finally, because of these specific limitations that are often inherent in qualitative research (Creswell, 2007), the results of this study can only be generalized to older African American lesbian women and gay men within this study.

FUTURE DIRECTIONS

As people of color, older African American participants may have different perspectives than older Caucasian people of European descent who benefit from privilege based on skin color (McIntosh, 1999). Therefore, a natural study for further research would be separate qualitative studies based on the gender of older African American lesbian women and gay men to explore possible differences based on gender, and a quantitative study comparing the aging experiences of African American lesbian women and gay men with African American heterosexual men and women. A qualitative, Phenomenological study specifically capturing the lived experiences of African American bisexual and transgender individuals would increase the knowledge of a segment of the African American population that is rarely studied. Other research could include examining the constructs of religious and spiritual beliefs among all LGBT sexual identities including African Americans is vital to further understanding this population and providing solutions as they move into old age. These studies would add to the knowledge initiated in this study in regard to the culture and the viable outreach methods for this population as well as to inform federal and state policy makers on the increased risks older African American LGBT individuals face without federal and marital benefits and employment and other legal protections. Additional research may be able to make recommendations to include older African American lesbian women and gay men in the aging-successfully discussions germane to policy, housing, health care, and social and community services (Grant, 2010).

NOTES

1. In this article, "Black" and "African American" are used interchangeably.

2. Level I is comprised of raw data obtained through the dialogue from the interviews and answers to the survey instrument.

3. In the Level II process, the researcher conducted an analysis and interpretation of the data that reflected the data synthesized from the communication nuances of the participants to a more psychological scientific language (Giorgi, 1997).

REFERENCES

American Association of Retired Persons. (2010). *At a glance fact book.* 2010: 50+ (Internal document). Washington, DC: Author.

Azibo, D. (1989). Mental health and nosology of Black/African personality disorder. *The Journal of Black Psychology, 15*(2), 175–178.

Beedon, L., & Wu, K. B. (2004). *African Americans age 65 and older: Their sources of income.* Washington, DC: AARP Public Policy Institute.

Cahill, S., South, K., & Spade, J. (2000). *Outing age: Public policy issues affecting gay, lesbian, bisexual and transgender elders.* Washington, DC: National Gay and Lesbian Task Force Policy Institute. Retrieved from http://www.lgbthealth.net/downloads/research/NGLTFoutingage.pdf

Collins, P. H. (2000). *Black feminist thought: Knowledge, consciousness and the politics of empowerment* (2nd ed.). New York, NY: Routledge.

Creswell, J. (2007). *Qualitative inquiry and research and research design: Choosing among five approaches.* Thousand Oaks, CA: Sage.

Currey, R. (2008). Ageism in health care: Time for a change. *Aging Well, 1*(1), 16–21. Retrieved from http://www.agingwellmag.com/archive/winter08p16.shtml

Fish, J. (2007). *Lesbian, gay and bisexual people from Black and minority ethnic communities*. London, England: Department of Health, Sexual Orientation and Gender Identity Advisory Group Work Program.

Fisher, A. (2007). Through colored glasses: The identity integration process of working class African American lesbian women (Doctoral dissertation). Alliant International University, San Francisco, CA. Retrieved from Proquest Dissertations & Theses (http://gradworks.umi.com/32/82/3282276.html)

Gabbay, S., & Wahler, J. (2002). Lesbian aging: Review of a growing literature. *Journal of Gay and Lesbian Social Services, 14*(3), 1–21.

Giorgi, A. (1997). The theory, practice, and evaluation of the phenomenological method as a qualitative research procedure. *Journal of Phenomenological Psychology, 28*(2), 25–260.

González, C. (2007). Age-graded sexualities: The struggles of our aging body. *Sexuality & Culture, 11*(4), 31–47.

Grant, J. (2010). *Outing Age 2010: Public policy issues affecting lesbian, gay, bisexual and transgender elders*. Washington, DC: National Gay and Lesbian Task Force Policy Institute. Retrieved from http://www.thetaskforce.org

Grasswick, H. (2006). Feminist social epistemology. *Stanford Encyclopedia of Psychology*. Retrieved from http://plato.stanford.edu/entries/feminist-social-epistemology

Kertzner, R., Meyer, I., Frost, D., & Stirratt, M. (2009). Social and psychological well-being in lesbian women, gay men and bisexuals: The effects of race, gender and sexual identity. *American Journal of Orthopsychiatry, 79*, 500–510.

Kostere, K., Kostere, S., & Percy, B. (2009). *Qualitative analysis Parts I–III: Residencies learning activity workbook, Track 3*. Minneapolis, MN: Capella University.

McIntosh, P. (1999). *White privilege: Unpacking the invisible knapsack* (Working Paper No. 189). Wellesley, MA: Wellesley College Center for Research on Women. Retrieved from http://www.iub.edu/~tchsotl/part2/McIntosh%20White%20Privilege.pdf

Moradi, B., Wiseman, M., DeBlaere, C., Sarkees, A., Goodman, M., Brewster, M., & Huang, Y. (2010). LGB of color and White individuals' perception of heterosexist stigma, internalized homophobia and outness: Comparison of levels and links. *Counseling Psychologist, 38*, 397–424.

National Gay and Lesbian Task Force. (2009). *Aging: Reports and research*. Washington, DC: Author. Retrieved from http://www.thetaskforce.org/issues/aging

Neville, H., Coleman, M., Falconer, J., & Holmes, D. (2005). Color-blind racial ideology and psychological false consciousness among African Americans. *Journal of Black Psychology, 31*(1), 27–45.

Pope, M., Wierzalia, E., Barret, B., & Rankin, M. (2007). Sexual intimacy issues for aging gay men. *Adultspan Journal, 6*(2), 68–82.

Smith, C. (2007). Queer as Black folk? *Wisconsin Law Review, 2*, 380–407. Retrieved from http://wisconsinlawreview.org/wp-content/files/5-Smith.pdf

Strom, R., Carter, T., & Schmidt, K. (2004). African Americans in senior settings: On the need for educating grandparents. *Educational Gerontology, 30,* 287–303.

Szymanski, D., & Gupta, A. (2009). Examining the relationship between multiple internalized oppressions and African American, lesbian, gay, bisexual and questioning persons' self-esteem and psychological distress. *Journal of Counseling Psychology, 56,* 110–118.

U.S. Census Bureau. (2012). *USA: People QuickFacts.* Washington, DC: Author. Retrieved from http://quickfacts.census.gov/qfd/states/00000.html

Wilson, B., & Miller, R. (2002). Strategies for managing heterosexism used among African American gay and bisexual men. *Journal of Black Psychology, 28,* 371–391.

Woody, I. (2008, March). *Lift every voice: An analysis of the impact of race, ethnicity, gender, socioeconomic status and sexuality on the health and economic well being of older women of African descent, including women who partner with women.* Poster session presented at the annual meeting of American Society on Aging, Washington, DC.

Woolf, L. (1998). *Gay and lesbian aging.* Webster Groves, MO: Webster University. Retrieved from http://www.webster.edu/~woolflm/oldergay.html

Service Utilization Among Older Adults With HIV: The Joint Association of Sexual Identity and Gender

MARK BRENNAN-ING, PhD

AIDS Community Research Initiative of America (ACRIA), ACRIA Center on HIV & Aging, New York, New York; New York University College of Nursing, New York, New York, USA

LIZ SEIDEL, MSW

AIDS Community Research Initiative of America (ACRIA), ACRIA Center on HIV & Aging, New York, New York, USA

ANDREW S. LONDON, PhD

Department of Sociology, LGBT Studies Program, Gerontology Center, Center for Policy Research, & Center for Aging and Policy Studies, Syracuse University, Syracuse, New York, New York, USA

SEAN CAHILL, PhD

Gay Men's Health Crisis (GMHC), Wagner School of Public Service, New York University, New York, New York, USA

STEPHEN E. KARPIAK, PhD

AIDS Community Research Initiative of America (ACRIA), ACRIA Center on HIV & Aging, New York, New York, USA

This study examines the association of sexual identity and gender among older clients with HIV at an AIDS service organization using the Andersen Model. Data confirm those aging with HIV exhibit high rates of age-associated illnesses 10 to 20 years before expected. They have fragile social networks that cannot supply the informal supports needed. This aging population will need to increasingly access community-based services. Sexual identity and gender were weak covariates of service utilization. Although heterosexual men used more services, utilization was largely predicted by service needs and the use of case management. Implications for service delivery and policy are discussed.

Few are aware that the number of people 50 years and older living with HIV/AIDS (OPLWHA) has nearly doubled since 2001 (Centers for Disease Control and Prevention [CDC], 2008). The success of antiretroviral therapies has transformed HIV into a manageable chronic illness. People living with HIV can now expect a marked increase in life expectancy (Walensky et al., 2006). As a result, adults 50 years and older will comprise fully one-half of those living with this disease by 2015 in the United States (Effros et al., 2008). But, there are complications associated with this success. There is mounting evidence that OPLWHA, most being between the ages of 50 and 60 years, are experiencing high rates of comorbid illnesses 2 decades earlier than their non-infected peers. They report three times as many comorbid conditions as community-dwelling adults 70 years and older (Havlik, 2009; Havlik, Brennan, & Karpiak, 2011).

Older adults typically turn to family for needed assistance in coping with the challenges of aging, including illness (Cantor & Brennan, 2000). However, the majority of OPLWHA have fragile, friend-centered informal social networks, and many of these friends are also living with HIV (Cantor, Brennan, & Karpiak, 2009; Shippy & Karpiak, 2005a, 2005b). Without support from their informal networks, OPLWHA will increasingly need to access formal, community-based services as they age (Brennan, Strauss, & Karpiak, 2010). Although research has examined the use and integration of informal and formal care among the HIV population (London et al., 2001; London, LeBlanc, & Aneshensel, 1998), the extent to which these findings can be generalized to OPLWHA is uncertain, as they are based on data from earlier periods of the epidemic using primarily younger samples.

The face of HIV is also changing. Although initially considered by many to be primarily a disease of gay men, the epidemic has increasingly affected heterosexual men and women in low-income, minority communities (Karpiak & Brennan, 2009). In response to this demographic shift, AIDS service organizations, many of which emerged out of the post-Stonewall network of gay community-based health and social service organizations have had to broaden their focus. Originally these organizations almost exclusively served the gay, lesbian, bisexual, and transgender (GLBT) community. Now these organizations have had to broaden their focus in order to serve everyone, regardless of sexual identity and make special efforts to meet the needs of HIV-positive heterosexual adults.

The purpose of this study is to examine the joint association of sexual identity and gender in terms of service utilization among OPLWHA who were recent clients of a large AIDS service organization in New York City. By studying OPLWHA who have connections to a major AIDS service organization, we are likely identifying OPLWHA who have more needs, but also more access to community-based resources and formal services—that is, these agencies often serve as points-of-entry into the larger system of AIDS-specific and more general social services (Bettencourt, Hodgins, Huba, & Pickett, 1998). Documenting variations in service use that are driven by health needs is important for policy, program planning, and development. Examining variations in service use driven by factors other than needs, such as sexual identity, is needed as it reflects inequitable access (Andersen, 1995; Institute of Medicine [IOM], 2011) and can provide the impetus for recommendations about changes in policies and programs that aim to redress such inequity.

SERVICE UTILIZATION AMONG OLDER ADULTS

Theoretical and empirical work in social gerontology points to an increasing reliance on formal community-based services as people age, due to growing service needs that cannot be met by their informal network of family, friends, and neighbors. The availability of instrumental and emotional support is closely tied to the viability of the informal social network, which helps to ensure the adequate care of people who are growing older (Cantor & Brennan, 2000). However, as people age, their social networks become smaller due to the loss of significant others, illness, and changing social roles (e.g., retirement). Cantor's *Hierarchical Compensatory Theory* of social supports contends that when people need assistance they prefer kin, first turning to close family such as spouses and children (Cantor & Mayer, 1978). When these individuals are not available, more distant relatives, friends, and neighbors are engaged. When these latter supports are not available, formal services are accessed. Formal services are also utilized when the capacity of informal caregivers is exceeded by the needs of the older adult, for example, when advanced medical care in the home is required (Cantor & Brennan, 2000).

The Hierarchical Compensatory Theory is supported by research on a range of older populations. Cantor and Brennan (1993) found that 56% of older adults in New York City had turned to one formal service in the last year and those who used more services tended to live alone, were in poorer health, and had lower incomes. Other studies report that many older socially isolated adults in the general population consider religious congregations, a source of community-based supports, to be their "surrogate families" and the foundation of their social networks (Sheehan, Wilson, & Marella, 1988; Tirrito & Choi, 2005). With regard to OPLWHA, their reliance on friends as the mainstay of their social networks compensates for the absence of a spouse/partner and the relative scarcity of kin (Brennan et al., 2010; Shippy & Karpiak, 2005a, 2005b). It is noteworthy that, although this type of friend-centered network has been typical of older GLBT adults, as described later, the same pattern is observed among heterosexual OPLWHA (Cantor et al., 2009). Given this paucity of informal social network resources, one could hypothesize that OPLWHA will need to access formal community-based services to meet their needs.

SERVICE USE IN THE OLDER GLBT COMMUNITY

Like OPLWHA, older GLBT adults rely on friend-centered social networks consisting of so-called families of choice, rather than biological families of origin (Shippy, Cantor, & Brennan, 2004). Therefore, it is friends who are more likely than family to provide assistance with tasks like caregiving for older GLBT adults. In this population, those who have friends available to provide assistance do better on measures of mental health compared to their peers without such resources (Masini & Barrett, 2008; Shippy et al., 2004; Smith, McCaslin, Chang, Martinez, & McGrew, 2010). However, the absence of blood ties between helpers from the family of choice and the older GLBT adult can have negative consequences; interactions with the biological family can often be negative and problematic and the lack of legal recognition of same-sex partners can result in their exclusion from making caregiving decisions (Cantor, Brennan, & Shippy, 2004). The literature on formal service utilization among older GLBT adults is extremely limited. In addition, most studies on service utilization in the larger GLBT community that contain older adults in their samples do not include age in their analyses (IOM, 2011). GLBT individuals must often access services in unwelcoming environments, where staff lack knowledge about the GBLT community and consideration is not given to the sexual orientation or gender identity of clients (Bell, Bern-Klug, Kramer, & Saunders, 2010). In some instances, providers may exhibit negative attitudes toward GLBT individuals (Tan, 2005). The limited studies on the experiences of aging GLBT adults seeking services has documented a range of barriers that trace their origins to a dominant heterosexist culture that is intrinsically neither inclusive nor welcoming of this population. This is evidenced by assumptions of heterosexuality by providers, a lack of recognition of same sex partners, and discrimination from providers and heterosexual peers (Brotman, Ryan, & Cormier, 2003; Hughes, 2007). These barriers limit access to services and result in concomitantly higher levels of unmet service needs (Tjepkema, 2008). This body of work concludes that GLBT adults, including those who are older, may utilize fewer community-services when compared to their heterosexual peers due to access barriers, fear of discrimination, and unequal treatment on the part of service providers.

SERVICE UTILIZATION AMONG HIV-POSITIVE ADULTS

Research on service-seeking among adults living with HIV, many of whom are also sexual minorities, is limited. There are few documented differences in barriers to service between older and younger HIV-positive adults; older adults have generally lived longer with the disease and are, therefore, knowledgeable and skilled in accessing available HIV and related services (Fritsch, 2005). With regard to race/ethnicity, Basta, Shacham, and Reece (2008) found that African Americans tended to be "moderately engaged" in HIV-associated mental health care and are more likely to have taken part in recent substance abuse treatment as compared with Caucasians. In terms of sexual identity, Penniman et al. (2007) reported that most utilization differences based on sexual identity or gender did not remain significant after controlling for socioeconomic factors. It is unclear from the extant literature to what extent having a connection to an organization with strong ties to the GLBT community enhances service utilization among OPLWHA who are GLBT, or inhibits it among their non-GLBT peers.

A CONCEPTUAL FRAMEWORK FOR UNDERSTANDING SERVICE UTILIZATION

R. M. Andersen (1968, 1995) proposed a model to explain differential use of health services based on predisposing, enabling, and need factors. Predisposing factors comprise demographic, social, and cultural characteristics including race/ethnicity, education, and knowledge and beliefs about health care. Such factors influence individuals to seek (or not seek) formal services to help them address their health problems. Andersen described enabling factors as community and personal resources that facilitate service use, such as whether services exist in the community, if people know where to get the services and if they can afford them. Barriers to care are also included in this domain because they can inhibit, rather than promote, the use of services. Need for care is determined by health factors that affect the volume of health services used such as the number and severity of health conditions. Conceptually, need factors should be the primary engine of health and social service utilization.

However, although need should drive service utilization on the conceptual level, access to case management services may be equally important in understanding service utilization among people living with HIV in a fragmented and complex service delivery environment (London et al., 1998). Case management provides a variety of supports and functions as a metaservice that provides a bridge to other HIV and non-HIV community-based resources. W. E. Cunningham, Wong, and Hays (2008) found that those who utilize case management are more likely to have lower incomes and education, to be uninsured or publicly insured, to have a history of drug use, and to be racial/ethnic minorities, women, or heterosexuals. Similarly, Basta et al. (2008) found Blacks and Latinos were more likely to have recently accessed case management, compared to Whites, although the authors did not control for socioeconomic differences. The benefits of case management, such as increasing the likelihood of seeing a health care provider, more medical visits, and improvements in health outcomes for those with HIV that have not initiated antiretroviral treatment are supported by empirical data (Anthony et al., 2007; W. E. Cunningham et al., 2008).

The Andersen Model (Andersen, 1968, 1995) has been applied to numerous studies of healthcare and other types of service utilization in a variety of populations, including people living with HIV. Cantor and Brennan (1993) in examing formal service use among older adults in New York City found that the predisposing characteristics of increased age, lower socioeconomic status, living alone and being non-Latino were associated with greater utilization. Four enabling factors were positively associated with greater service use; connection to the entitlement system (defined as receiving Supplemental Security Income, Medicaid, or food stamps), having a small social network, being a caregiver, and involvement with neighbors (considered to be sources of information and linkages to the larger community). With regard to need factors, the perceived number of service needs predicted greater utilization. A study of people with HIV that predated the current antiretroviral era and used the Andersen Model framework found that predisposing factors such as being a racial/ethnic minority, or having low income or education were related to lower utilization of mental health outpatient care, but greater use of outpatient substance abuse care (Burnam et al., 2001).

Purpose and Rationale

The burgeoning population of older adults with HIV will increasingly turn to formal community-based services in the near future, given their high levels of health comorbidities and lack of informal social support. There is a dearth of research on the service utilization patterns of this aging population, resulting in the need to develop an evidence base for policy makers and program planners to begin to address this emerging issue. Gay and bisexual men are no longer the predominant group affected by HIV in many parts of the United States, and AIDS service organizations have needed to modify their programs to be inclusive of heterosexuals and women. There is evidence that GLBT individuals may underutilize health and social services, but it is not clear if this is the case among those who are growing older with HIV. This study is based on an assessment of OPLWHA that identified service needs resulting from physical and mental problems, as well as expressed need for services in the previous year. We examined how the joint association of sexual identity and gender was related to both needs and service utilization among older adults with HIV to provide information for policymakers and program recommendations to better serve this population.

METHOD

Sample

Data for this study were obtained from a convenience sample of adults 50 years and older, who had received services at Gay Men's Health Crisis (GMHC), one of the largest AIDS service organizations in New York City in the 6 months prior to data collection. Eligibility criteria were being age 50 years and older, being English-speaking, and being without any cognitive deficits, in the judgment of the research assistant, that would preclude participation. Out of the 205 surveys that were obtained, 25 were incomplete resulting in a final sample of 180. The average age of the sample was 55.5 years, and most (80%) were between ages 50 and 60 years old. Almost, three-fourths of the sample were men (78%), 22% were women, and no one identified as transgender. Over one-half of the participants self-identified as gay or lesbian (55%), 15% as bisexual, and 30% as heterosexual. There were significant gender differences in sexual identity. Most men identified as homosexual (65%), followed by heterosexual (19%) and bisexual (16%). Among women, 75% identified as heterosexual, 16% as lesbian, and 9% as bisexual.

Measures

The survey instrument was adapted from the Research on Older Adults with HIV (ROAH) study (Brennan, Karpiak, Shippy, & Cantor, 2009), and covered a range of issues that included health, functional ability, social supports, caregiving, and use of formal community-based services. Details of the specific measures used in this article are described in the following.

Formal service utilization. Questions about services accessed in the previous year, in addition to those received at GMHC, were adapted from previous studies of service utilization among older New Yorkers (Cantor & Brennan, 2000). The time frame of the previous year was retained so as to facilitate comparisons between the study sample and comparison data. Four categories were assessed: *government agencies/offices* (e.g., Medicaid), *HIV/AIDS-related services* (e.g., HIV day program), *health/long-term care services* (e.g., emergency room), and *other older adult services* (e.g., senior center). The number of services used within each of the four categories and overall was summed to create variables indicating the total number of services used and the number used in each domain.

Sexual identity and gender. Respondents were asked to indicate their sexual identity (i.e., heterosexual, homosexual, or bisexual) and gender (i.e., male, female, male-to-female transgender, and female-to-male transgender).

Predisposing factors. Single items obtained information on *age, race, Hispanic origin, level of education,* and *history of incarceration.* Participants were asked how they became infected with HIV (anal sex, vaginal sex, sharing needles, other, or not sure), with sharing needles considered a proxy for *history of intravenous drug use* (IDU).

Enabling factors. Participants were asked about their current living arrangements (alone, with partner/spouse, with others) to assess the proportion *living alone. Level of assistance from the informal network* was assessed by whether participants had received any of eight types of social support from family and friends/neighbors, respectively. Questions on the types of support received were obtained from previous large-scale studies of older adults (Cantor & Brennan, 2000; Cantor et al., 2004).These types of support included instrumental help (i.e., shop/run errands, keep house/prepare meals, take or drive you places, help with mail/correspondence, and manage money/pay bills) and emotional support (i.e., provide advice on big decisions, talk when feeling low/need cheering up, and talk about personal/private matters). Each group of items was summed to create an index of overall family and friend support (range = 0–16). Participants were asked which of the following types of *insurance* they currently received (i.e., Medicaid, Medicare, or private insurance). Finally, participants were asked if they had used *case management* services in the prior year.

Need factors. Single-items assessed the *length of time since HIV diagnosis* and *prior AIDS diagnosis.* Participants were asked if they had experienced any of 27 physical and mental health conditions in the previous year, including HIV-related conditions (e.g., neuropathy), age-related conditions (e.g., sensory loss), chronic/terminal illnesses (e.g., diabetes and cancer), and mental or neurological disorders (e.g., depression). The number of *health comorbidities* was calculated by summing the positive responses to these items. The 10-item version of the Center for Epidemiological Studies Depression Scale (CES–D) was used to assess *depressive symptoms* (Andersen, Malmgren, Carter, & Patrick, 1994; Radloff, 1977). Participants were asked about the frequency of depressive symptoms experienced over the past week (none, a little, some, or most days). Responses were summed with higher scores indicating greater levels of depressive symptoms. Two items (e.g., "I was happy") are reverse scored. Inter-item reliability for this scale in this sample was high ($\alpha = .84$). Participants indicated their need for any of 11 types of services in the past year including instrumental help (e.g., housekeeping or personal care), long-term care (e.g., visiting nurse), and emotional support (e.g., personal or family counseling; see Table 1 for the complete list). Positive responses were summed to obtain the *number of service needs in the past year*. These items were obtained from previous large-scale studies of older adults (Cantor & Brennan, 2000).

Procedure

The study protocoland survey instrument were approved by the Copernicus Group Independent Review Board. Participants were recruited on-site at GMHC through flyers, referrals from program staff, and in-person through tabling during the meal/nutrition program hours in an area outside of the dining room. Those agreeing to participate were directed to a location on a different floor where they were met by research staff and seated in individual cubicles for privacy. Research staff obtained informed consent, and participants completed the self-administered survey on hardcopies ($n = 175$) or computer using Survey Monkey® ($n = 30$). Informed consent and survey completion lasted from 45 to 60 min. Following survey completion, participants were debriefed, thanked, and given a movie pass for their participation ($10 value). Due to the nature of recruitment and data collection, a response rate cannot be calculated.

Design and Analysis

This study used a correlational design to examine the covariates of service utilization among OPLWHA. The primary independent variable was sexual identity (i.e., heterosexual, homosexual, or bisexual). However, because differences in sexual identity were not equally distributed by gender in this sample (i.e., a preponderance of men were gay and bisexual, whereas women were predominantly heterosexual), we felt it was important to examine the joint association of these factors in our analysis. This entailed creating separate groups based both on sexual identity and gender. Because the number of lesbian and bisexual women was small (five and three, respectively), these individuals were excluded from analyses. In addition, 17 respondents were dropped because they did not report their sexual identity ($n = 16$) or gender ($n = 1$). Thus, our analytic sample included 155 participants in the following four groups; homosexual men ($n = 85$), bisexual men ($n = 21$), heterosexual men ($n = 25$), and heterosexual women ($n = 24$).

These four groups were used in bivariate analyses to examine differences regarding predisposing, enabling, need and service utilization variables, employing chi-square analysis for categorical/ordinal variables and analysis of variance for continuous measures. Prior to multivariate analyses, a bivariate correlational analysis was conducted to develop parsimonious

TABLE 1 Sample Descriptives and Service Use Covariates by Sexual and Gender Identity (Valid Percentages)

Variable	Total	Homosexual Men	Bisexual Men	Heterosexual Men	Heterosexual Women
Predisposing factors					
Age group*					
50–55 years	60.1	59.5	40.0	56.5	79.2
56–60 years	20.2	16.5	45.0	21.7	16.7
61+	19.6	24.1	15.0	21.7	4.2
Race/ethnicity***					
Non-Hispanic Black	33.3	20.0	61.9	56.0	50.0
Non-Hispanic White	30.0	43.5	19.0	20.0	12.5
Hispanic	27.2	32.9	9.5	24.0	33.3
All others	9.4	3.5	9.5	0.0	4.2
Highest education					
Less than high school	10.9	9.5	0.0	8.7	12.5
High school degree	18.9	15.5	23.8	21.7	25.0
Some college	34.9	29.8	47.6	39.1	45.8
College graduate/postgraduate	35.4	45.2	28.6	30.4	16.7
Ever been incarcerated (yes)***	28.2	12.9	35.0	60.0	39.1
How infected with HIV***					
Anal sex	45.9	74.1	38.1	8.0	1.0
Vaginal sex	26.2	3.7	9.5	52.0	73.9
Sharing needles	7.0	0.0	23.8	12.0	4.3
Other/multiple risks	21.0	22.2	28.6	28.0	17.4
Enabling factors					
Live alone (yes)	74.4	77.6	81.0	68.0	70.8
Benefits and insurance coverage					
Medicare**	45.7	52.4	61.9	40.0	17.4
Medicaid***	70.1	58.8	76.2	88.0	95.7
Private health Insurance**	20.7	31.8	14.3	8.0	8.7
Case management (yes)	51.5	44.4	70.0	58.3	59.1
Need factors					
Diagnosed with AIDS (yes)*	55.7	69.0	47.6	54.2	37.5

(Continued)

TABLE 1 (Continued)

Variable	Total	Homosexual Men	Bisexual Men	Heterosexual Men	Heterosexual Women
CES–D depressive symptoms					
Not depressed	47.9	45.6	42.1	52.0	43.5
Moderately depressed	17.6	11.4	15.8	24.0	30.4
Severely depressed	34.5	43.0	42.1	24.0	26.1
Need for services in the past year					
Meals brought to the home*	22.4	15.3	31.6	12.5	37.5
Housekeeping or personal care	22.9	19.0	26.3	20.8	29.2
Help with home repairs	28.6	26.2	42.1	20.8	33.3
Help finding a job	28.2	29.4	45.0	12.5	25.0
Personal or family counseling**	41.7	52.9	25.0	25.0	30.4
Care after hospital stay	24.4	24.7	21.1	8.7	33.3
Escort to doctor/clinic	30.6	28.2	26.3	29.2	33.3
Someone to call/visit regularly	31.1	31.0	30.0	21.7	39.1
Visiting nurse/home health aid	13.2	7.1	25.0	8.7	18.2
Help with entitlements	40.7	44.0	40.0	34.8	39.1
Place to socialize/meet people	53.6	58.3	65.0	43.5	43.5
	M (SD)	*M (SD)*	*M (SD)*	*M (SD)*	*M (SD)*
Predisposing factors					
Age	55.6 (5.8)	56.0 (6.2)	56.8 (5.7)	55.6 (5.9)	52.9 (3.0)
Enabling factors					
Family and friend support	3.6 (3.7)	3.4 (3.4)	2.9 (3.2)	3.6 (4.3)	4.7 (4.2)
Need factors					
Time since HIV diagnosis (months)	189.3 (73.1)	192.6 (76.1)	204.2 (67.8)	172.6 (72.8)	182.3 (67.2)
No. of comorbid conditions	3.4 (2.7)	3.5 (2.7)	4.1 (3.8)	3.0 (2.2)	2.5 (2.1)
CES–D depressive symptoms	11.3 (6.3)	12.0 (6.7)	11.7 (5.0)	9.5 (6.5)	10.3 (4.4)
No. of service needs	3.2 (2.7)	3.3 (2.6)	3.5 (2.6)	2.2 (2.4)	3.5 (3.2)

Note. N = 155: homosexual men (*n* = 85); bisexual men (*n* = 21); heterosexual men (*n* = 25); heterosexual women (*n* = 24). CES–D = Center for Epidemiological Studies Depression Scale.

*p < .05. **p < .01. ***p < .001.

regression models and to test for multicollinearity of covariates. Categorical variables were dummy-coded prior to correlational analysis. Covariates that were neither significantly correlated with the dependent variables (i.e., $p < .05$) nor considered important control variables were excluded from further analysis. Listwise deletion of missing variables was used for multivariate analysis, rendering an effective sample size of 122 for the service utilization regressions.

Multivariate analysis consisted of logistic regression for the dichotomous dependent variable (i.e., use of case management: yes or no) and ordinary least squares (OLS) regressions for continuous dependent variables (i.e., number of government offices and agencies, HIV/AIDS-related services, health and long-term care services, and "other" older adult services used). The same hierarchical method of entry of independent variables was used for both logistic and OLS regression analyses in accordance with the Andersen Model (Andersen, 1968, 1995). The first block of variables consisted of three of the four variables corresponding to the sexual identity/gender groups—namely, heterosexual men, heterosexual women, and bisexual men; homosexual men served as the reference group. Following this block, the predisposing, enabling, and need factor blocks were entered separately as described in the Andersen Model. Within each of these three blocks, a forward stepwise procedure of entry was used to ensure adequate statistical power given the listwise sample size. Regression models were evaluated in terms of the significance of the individual blocks and overall model (chi-square or F test), the significance of individual covariates (odds ratios or betas), and the amount of variance explained by the regression model. Diagnostics did not indicate any significant multicollinearity of covariates in the regression analyses.

RESULTS

Bivariate Analyses

Predisposing factors. The average age of this sample was 55.6, which did not differ significantly among the four sexual/gender identity groups. However, there were significantly higher proportions of individuals over the age of 60 among homosexual and heterosexual men (24% and 22%, respectively), as compared with bisexual men and heterosexual women (hereafter referred to as women), 15% and 4%, respectively. Race/ethnicity also significantly varied by group, with homosexual men most likely to be either non-Hispanic White or Hispanic (44% and 33%, respectively), as compared with the other three groups where the majority was non-Hispanic Black (see Table 1). Educational attainment did not differ significantly among the four groups, with over two-thirds reporting either some college (35%) or a college degree/postgraduate degree (35%). Homosexual men were significantly less likely to report a history of incarceration (13%) as compared to heterosexual men (60%), bisexual men (35%), or women (39%). When asked about how they had become infected with HIV, homosexual men were significantly more likely to report anal sex (74%), whereas vaginal sex was the primary mode of transmission among heterosexual men and women (52% and 74%, respectively). Bisexual men were the most likely to report being infected through sharing needles (24%), as compared to 12% or less in the other three groups.

Enabling factors. As shown in Table 1, the proportion living alone was substantial (74%) and did not differ significantly as a function of sexual identity/gender. With regard to assistance from the informal social network, participants reported receiving 3.6 types of help, on average, and this did not differ significantly by group. In terms of insurance coverage, bisexual men were the most likely to report being enrolled in Medicare (62%), followed by 52% of homosexual men and 40% of heterosexual men. Only 17% of women had Medicare coverage. In contrast, heterosexual men and women were the most likely to be enrolled in the Medicaid program (88% and 96%, respectively), followed by bisexual men (76%) and homosexual men (59%). Although nearly one-third of homosexual men reported private insurance coverage, this proportion dropped to 14% for bisexual men and approximately 8% of heterosexual men and women. Case management services were reported by over one-half (52%) of participants and did not differ significantly by sexual identity/gender.

Need factors. Homosexual men were the most likely to report having received a diagnosis of AIDS (i.e., CD-4 count ≤ 200 or opportunistic infection); 69% of homosexual men reported an AIDS diagnosis as compared to about one-half of those in the other two male groups and 38% of women (see Table 1). The average time since HIV diagnosis was 189 months (15.75 years), which did not differ significantly by sexual identity/gender. On average, older adults with HIV in this sample reported 3.4 comorbid conditions in addition to HIV with no significant group differences. A majority of the sample had at least moderate depressive symptoms; 35% reported a level of depressive symptoms on the CES–D indicative of severe depression, whereas 18% reported moderate levels of depressive symptoms. There were no significant group differences in CES–D scores. Few group differences emerged on service needs in the previous year. Overall, socialization needs were the most frequently mentioned (54%), followed by needing personal/family counseling (42%), and help accessing entitlement programs (41%). Other types of instrumental assistance needs (e.g., housekeeping, home repairs) were reported by 20% to 30% of participants, whereas visiting nurse/home health aides was the lowest reported need at 13%. Women and bisexual men were approximately twice as likely to need meals brought to them at home (38% and 32%, respectively) compared to homosexual or heterosexual

men (15% and 13%, respectively). The only other significant group difference to emerge was the need for personal/family counseling. Over one-half
of homosexual men reported needing this type of assistance as compared
with 30% or less for the other three groups. The average number of service
needs was 3.2 and did not differ by sexual identity/gender.

Formal service utilization. Among the government agencies and offices,
the New York City Human Resources Administration was the most frequently
utilized in the past year (66%), followed by the Social Security Office (62%).
Medicaid and Medicare offices were the next most frequently utilized (49%
and 35%, respectively; see Table 2). The New York City Housing Authority
(25%) and police department (20%) were more frequently utilized than either
the Veterans' Administration (VA; 12%) or New York City Department for the
Aging (9%). The low proportions using the latter agency was not surprising
given the relatively low proportion of persons age 60 and older in this sample. Among these services, bisexual men were the most likely to access the
Medicare Office (50%), followed by heterosexual men (44%) and homosexual men (35%), as compared with only 6% of women. Heterosexual men
were the most likely to access the VA/VA hospital (35%), as compared
to bisexual or homosexual men (16% and 8%, respectively) and women
(0%). There were no significant group differences in the average number of
government agencies and offices accessed in the previous year (2.5).

With regard to HIV/AIDS services, AIDS service organizations were the
most frequently mentioned provider and utilized by 88% of the sample. The
New York City HIV/AIDS Service Administration (HASA) followed, with 70%
of respondents turning to this agency. Participation in Housing Assistance
programs and HIV day programs was mentioned by over one-third of participants (36% and 36%, respectively). The use of AIDS service organizations
and Housing Assistance did not differ significantly by group; however, heterosexual men were the most frequent users of HASA and HIV day program
services. Nearly all of the heterosexual men in this sample used HASA (96%),
followed by bisexual men (85%), women (68%), and homosexual men (63%).
Over one-half of heterosexual men participated in HIV day programs (55%),
as did nearly as many women (48%). Use of day programs by homosexual and bisexual men was considerably lower (26% and 28%, respectively).
On average, participants accessed 2.2 HIV/AIDS services, and there were no
differences between the four groups.

The most frequently utilized health care service was the dentist/dental
clinic, reported by 61% of participants (see Table 2). Forty-four percent of
participants used mental/behavioral health services and 22% reported using
drug/alcohol treatment or recovery services. With regard to hospital use,
outpatient services were the most frequently reported (44%), followed by
the emergency room visits (40%) and inpatient hospital stays (23%). Thirty
percent reported receiving medical care from a private physician or clinic,

TABLE 2 Use of Services by Sexual and Gender Identity (Valid Percentages)

Variable	Total	Homosexual Men	Bisexual Men	Heterosexual Men	Heterosexual Women
Government agencies & offices					
Social Security	61.7	61.0	63.2	64.0	56.5
Medicaid	49.1	43.2	47.1	58.3	65.0
Medicare*	35.3	35.1	50.0	43.5	5.6
VA/VA Hospital**	12.2	8.2	15.8	34.8	0.0
NYC Human Resources Administration	65.9	60.0	80.0	70.8	77.3
NYC HA	24.7	23.0	21.1	30.4	35.0
NYC DFTA	8.7	6.8	5.9	17.4	0.0
Police department	20.0	12.0	27.8	22.7	31.6
HIV/AIDS services					
HIV day program*	35.5	26.3	27.8	54.5	47.6
Housing assistance for PLWHA	36.0	27.0	42.1	54.5	42.9
HASA**	69.8	62.5	85.0	95.5	68.2
AIDS service organization	88.0	94.0	85.7	91.3	87.0
Health/long-term care services					
Emergency room	39.9	35.4	50.0	52.2	40.9
Private medical clinic	30.1	36.6	15.0	33.3	15.8
HMO	18.4	19.5	10.0	27.3	5.6
Mental/behavioral health services	43.9	47.0	52.4	37.5	40.0
Drug/alcohol treatment or recovery*	22.3	14.8	21.1	39.1	36.8

Outpatient hospital	43.9	41.5	60.0	50.0	33.3
Inpatient hospital	22.6	20.0	20.0	30.4	29.4
Dentist or dental clinic	60.7	65.9	65.0	56.5	54.5
Home health care (all types)	16.5	12.0	10.0	30.4	19.0
Assisted living/long-term care facility*	5.0	2.4	0.0	22.7	5.0
Hospice	4.6	2.5	0.0	15.0	5.3
Other older adult services					
Senior center	17.4	15.6	10.5	30.4	15.0
Meal or nutrition program*	59.3	66.7	63.2	60.9	33.3
Self-help group	39.9	46.3	42.1	34.8	35.0
Clergy (minister, priest, rabbi, iman)	29.4	32.1	30.0	26.1	22.7
Legal services	40.5	43.0	47.6	37.5	40.9
	M (SD)	M (SD)	M (SD)	M (SD)	M (SD)
Number of government services	2.5 (1.8)	2.3 (1.8)	2.8 (1.7)	3.2 (2.0)	2.4 (1.4)
No. of HIV/AIDS services	2.2 (1.2)	2.0 (1.1)	2.3 (1.1)	2.6 (1.1)	2.3 (1.3)
No. of health/long-term care services	3.4 (2.7)	2.3 (2.5)	3.6 (2.0)	4.2 (3.6)	2.9 (2.6)
No. of other older adults services	1.8 (1.5)	1.9 (1.4)	1.8 (1.3)	1.8 (1.6)	1.3 (1.5)
Total no. of services	9.9 (5.1)	9.5 (4.9)	10.4 (4.1)	11.8 (5.8)	8.8 (5.1)

Note. $N = 155$: homosexual men ($n = 85$); bisexual men ($n = 21$); heterosexual men ($n = 25$); heterosexual women ($n = 24$). VA = Veterans' Administration; NYC = New York City; HA = Housing Authority; DFTA = Department for the Aging; PLWHA= people living with HIV/AIDS; HASA = HIV/AIDS Service Administration; HMO = health maintenance organization.

*$p < .05$. **$p < .01$.

whereas 18% received these services through a health maintenance organization. Long-term and end-of-life care was reported relatively infrequently, with 17% using any type of home health care, 5% using institutional long-term care or assisted living, and 5% using hospice care. There were few significant group differences in the use of health-related services, but similar to HIV/AIDS services, heterosexual men emerged as the more frequent service users. Heterosexual men were significantly more likely to report drug/alcohol treatment and recovery (39%), followed by women (37%), whereas 21% of bisexual men and 15% of homosexual men used these services. Heterosexual men also reported the greatest utilization of assisted living/long-term care facilities (23%), as compared with 5% of less of the other three groups. On average, participants used 3.4 health and long-term care services, and this did not differ significantly by group.

In terms of other older adult services, meal and nutrition programs were most often mentioned (59%), followed by legal services (41%). Nearly 40% reported using self-help groups. Seeking help from religious leaders was reported by almost one-third of the sample (29%), whereas senior center use was relatively infrequent (17%), likely due to the low proportion of the sample over the age of 60 (20%), which is the usual cutoff for accessing senior services. The only significant group difference in the use of these other services was in terms of meal and nutrition programs, which were accessed by approximately two-thirds of men, regardless of sexual identity. In contrast, only one-third of women reported using meal programs, which is in line with their greater expressed need for meals brought to them at home as noted earlier. Participants used 1.8 other older adult services, on average; and again, there were no significant group differences in this regard. Looking at all four groups of services (i.e., government agencies, HIV/AIDS, health/long-term care, and other older adult) participants reported using 9.9 services, on average, over the previous year with no significant group differences.

Multivariate Analyses

Prior to multivariate analysis, Pearson correlations of sexual identity/gender, predisposing, enabling, and need covariates with case management and service utilization variables were calculated. Predisposing factors were age, race/ethnicity, education, history of incarceration, and HIV infection through sharing needles (a proxy of history of IDU). Enabling characteristics were living alone, help from family and friends, insurance coverage (Medicare, Medicaid, or private insurance), and use of case management. Need factors were prior AIDS diagnosis, length of time since HIV diagnosis, number of comorbid conditions, CES–D depressive symptoms, and number of service needs in the past year. Table 3 shows the final list of covariates retained for the logistic and multiple regression models and their associated correlation

TABLE 3 Correlations of Covariates With Service Utilization Variables

Covariate	Case Management	Total Service	Government Agencies	HIV/AIDS Services	Health/Long-Term Care	Other Older Adult
Homosexual male	-.18*	-.07	-.14	-.18*	-.02	.10
Bisexual male	.14	.03	.05	.04	-.00	.01
Heterosexual male	.05	.17*	.17*	.18*	.12	-.01
Heterosexual female	.06	-.10	-.04	.03	-.09	-.15
Age	-.17*	-.04	.07	-.18*	-.06	.04
Black	.12	-.08	.08	-.01	-.11	-.18*
Latino	-.11	.09	.03	.08	.04	.12
Education	-.02	-.08	-.15	-.20*	.01	.05
Incarcerated	.09	.14	.14	.21**	.04	.06
IDU HIV infected	.14	.02	.11	-.02	.03	-.09
Total family/friend help	.13	.20**	-.04	.09	.26***	.21**
Medicare	-.03	.16	.19*	.02	.09	.12
Medicaid	.22**	.23**	.33***	.27***	.14	-.11
Private insurance	-.20**	-.16	-.23**	-.35***	.02	.01
Case manager	1.00	.46***	.31***	.37***	.39***	.17*
AIDS diagnosis	-.06	.05	.04	.02	-.02	.13
CES–D depressive symptoms	-.09	.23**	.18*	.05	.30***	-.00
No. of comorbid conditions	.21**	.36***	.24**	.18*	.37***	.13
No. of service needs	.19**	.31***	.09	.18*	.29***	.30***

Note. Pairwise *N* = 155. IDU = intravenous drug use; CES–D = Center for Epidemiological Studies Depression Scale.

*p < .05. **p < .01. ***p < .001.

TABLE 4 Logistic Regression on Use of Case Management Services Among Older Adults With HIV

Covariate	B	SE	OR	95% CI
Model 1[a]				
Heterosexual male	.47	.51	1.60	.59−4.31
Heterosexual female	.72	.54	2.06	.72−5.88
Bisexual male	1.06	.59	2.88	.91−9.10
Model 2[b]				
Heterosexual male	.39	.56	1.48	.50−4.41
Heterosexual female	.41	.59	1.50	.47−4.76
Bisexual male	.85	.62	2.34	.69−7.91
Medicaid	1.19	.48	3.30	1.29−8.43
No. of service needs	.23	.08	1.26	1.07−1.49

Note. Listwise $N = 123$. OR = odds ration; CI = confidence interval.
[a]$\chi^2(3, N = 123) = 4.62, p = .202$; Nagelkerke $R^2 = .05$. [b]$\chi^2(5, N =123) = 19.51, p < .005$; Nagelkerke $R^2 = .20$.

coefficients with the service use dependent variables. A prior AIDS diagnosis was retained as a control because of its conceptual importance to service use in this population. Although HIV infection through IDU was not correlated with service use, we retained this variable because past IDU was significantly higher among bisexual men, and could have played a role in current need for services. Living alone and length of time since HIV diagnosis were not significantly correlated with any of the service utilization variables and were not retained for multivariate analysis.

Logistic regression on case management use. As shown in Table 3, the enabling factor of the use of case management services was significantly correlated with four of the five service use variables. We conducted a binary logistic regression on the use of case management services utilizing the sexual identity/gender dummy-coded variables in the first block, followed by the predisposing, enabling, and need factor components of the Andersen Model (Andersen, 1968, 1995) for the other service utilization variables in the second block (see Table 4). Sexual identity/gender was not related to the use of case management when either entered separately or in combination with the other factors. No predisposing factors were significant in the case management logistic regression; however, use of case management was significantly related to enabling and need factors. Being enrolled in Medicaid increased the odds of case management use by over three and one-third times. Of the need factors, only the number of service needs retained its significance in multivariate analysis, with 26% greater odds of case management use for each need reported. The final model chi-square was significant and explained 20% of the variance in case management utilization.

Multiple regressions on service utilization. Table 5 displays the results of the multiple regressions on service utilization. In terms of sexual identity/gender, being a heterosexual man was related to greater total service

TABLE 5 Andersen Model Regressions on Total Services, and Government, HIV/AIDS, Health-Related Services, and Other Community-Based Services

Covariate	Total β	Total SE	Total p	Government β	Government SE	Government p	HIV/AIDS β	HIV/AIDS SE	HIV/AIDS p	Health-Related β	Health-Related SE	Health-Related p	Other β	Other SE	Other p
Step 1															
Heterosexual men	.18	.99	.02	.10	.43	.25	.16	.26	.05	.12	.50	.15	.04	.34	.67
Heterosexual women	-.04	1.04	.57	-.06	.47	.48	-.03	.27	.74	-.08	.52	.30	-.16	.35	.08
Bisexual men	-.02	1.06	.76	-.02	.46	.81	-.02	.28	.81	-.02	.54	.81	-.02	.36	.84
Step 2 (predisposing)															
Education							-.21	.10	.01						
Step 3 (enabling)															
Help from family/friends	.13	.73	.08							.15	.05	.07	.13	.04	.16
Medicare				.18	.31	.04									
Medicaid				.27	.37	.003									
Private insurance				.30	.31	.001	-.25	.24	.003						
Case manager	.45	.74	.001				.27	.20	.001	.34	.37	.001	.16	.25	.07
Step 4 (Need):															
CES–D	.23	.06	.003	.18	.02	.03				.33	.03	.001	.31	.05	.001
No. of needs	.26	.14	.001				.25	.04	.003	.22	.08	.009			

Note. Listwise $N = 122$. Total services: $F(7, 115) = 11.89, p < .001$; total $R^2 = .42$. Government services: $F(7, 115) = 6.41, p < .001$; total $R^2 = .28$. HIV/AIDS services: $F(7, 122) = 8.37, p < .001$; total $R^2 = .34$. Health services: $F(7, 115) = 9.57, p < .001$; total $R^2 = .33$. Other older adults services: $F(6, 116) = 4.95, p < .001$; total $R^2 = .20$. CES–D = Center for Epidemiological Studies Depression Scale.

use. None of the predisposing factors was significantly related to total service utilization. Of the enabling factors, being enrolled in Medicare and utilization of case management were both significant positive covariates of total service use. Considering need factors, depressive symptoms and the number of service needs in the previous year were significantly and positively related to the total number of services used. The regression model explained 42% of the variance in overall service utilization.

With regard to government offices and agencies, we did not find significant differences in the use of these services based on sexual identity/gender nor were there any significant predisposing factors that were related to this domain of service utilization. Of the enabling factors, being enrolled in either Medicaid or Medicare was positively related to use of government services, which was not surprising given that the Medicare and Medicaid offices were two of the agencies in this group. The enabling factor of case management was also a significant positive covariate of accessing offices and services provided by the government. Of the need factors, only higher levels of depressive symptoms were related to greater use of these services in the regression model, and explained 28% of the variance.

The regression model on HIV/AIDS service utilization explained 34% of the variance. Utilization of HIV/AIDS services was significantly related to sexual identity/gender, with heterosexual men using greater numbers of these services, even after controlling for the predisposing, enabling and need factors in the Andersen Model (Andersen, 1968, 1995). In terms of predisposing factors, greater education was negatively related to the utilization of HIV/AIDS services. In the block of enabling factors, having private insurance was negatively related to service use in this domain, whereas case management was a positive predictor of HIV/AIDS service use. Among the need factors, the number of service needs in the past year was significantly related to using a greater number of services from HIV/AIDS providers.

Use of health and long-term care services was not significantly related to sexual identity/gender, nor was the use of these services significantly related to predisposing factors. The enabling factor of help from family and friends was significant in this area when first entered into the model, but did not retain its significance when the remaining variables were entered. However, use of case management was significantly and positively related to greater use of health and long-term care services (see Table 5). Two of the need factors, the level of depressive symptoms and the number of services need in the past year, were significantly and positively related to greater use of these types of services. The regression model on health and long-term care services explained 33% of the variance in such utilization.

In the final group of other older adult services, sexual/gender identity again failed to emerge as a significant covariate of service use, and predisposing factors were not significantly related to greater use of these services. Of the enabling factors, help from family and friends was significant when entered into the model, but did not retain its significance when the need factors were entered in the following block. Of the need factors, the number of service needs was positively related to a greater use of other older adult services, and the final regression model explained 20% of the variance in older adult service use (see Table 5).

DISCUSSION

This study confirms prior research showing that this aging HIV population is exhibiting the early onset of multiple comorbid illnesses, with an average of three or more illnesses in addition to HIV/AIDS (Havlik, 2009; Havlik et al., 2011). Like prior research, there were high rates of depressive symptoms in this sample of OPLWHA, with 35% classified as severely depressed and 18% as moderately depressed. The burden of disease for this population whose average age is 56 years is substantial, and presages the need for ongoing informal supports and formal social services as they age. Similar to Penniman et al. (2007), we observed few differences in service utilization by sexual identity/gender when controlling for multiple factors. This lack of group differences regarding service utilization can be ascribed to the fact that, regardless of sexual identify or gender, most are experiencing the effects of HIV/AIDS, as well as high levels of depressive symptoms and multiple cormorbid illnesses. Minority sexual identity has been linked to lack of access and underutilization of services in the larger GLBT population (Brotman et al., 2003; Tjepkema, 2008). However, the health consequences of living with HIV/AIDS may be large enough to overshadow potential differences arising from sexual identity/gender as evidenced in this study. Thus, the experience of living and aging with HIV can be described as the great equalizer. It may also be that having a recent connection to GMHC, an AIDS service organization tasked with meeting the needs of a diverse clientele may have facilitated access to other community-based services by serving as a point-of-entry to other HIV and non-HIV services (Bettencourt et al., 1998). These findings also suggest that for this population aging with HIV in New York City, there is relatively equitable access to community-based services.

One difference emerges; heterosexual men used more services overall, and utilized more HIV-related services when compared to the other groups. However, the source of health insurance, an enabling factor, was significantly related to utilization, and may partly explain differences in the level of utilization associated with sexual identity/gender. Medicaid enrollment was significantly higher among heterosexual men and women compared to gay and bisexual men. Although we do not know the length of Medicaid enrollment, those who participated in this program prior to their HIV diagnosis may have a better understanding of how to access needs-based entitlements, which could be generalized to accessing HIV/AIDS services. In contrast, gay and bisexual men were more likely to be enrolled in Medicare or have private insurance coverage than their heterosexual peers. Having private insurance was negatively related to use of HIV-related services. Because those with private insurance likely have more economic resources than those who do not have such coverage, those with private insurance may be having their needs met from fee-for-service and other providers outside of the HIV service system. Medicaid and Medicare enrollment, which can facilitate connections to the larger array of entitlement programs and government support (Cantor & Brennan, 1993), was related to greater use of services overall and government agencies/offices in particular, and further illustrates how these programs serve as a point of entry to the formal service system.

However, the greatest contribution of enabling factors to service utilization was the use of case management. These results are similar to those of Ohl, Landon, Clearly, and LeMaster (2008), who found that PLWHA using on-site case management were more likely to exhibit a greater continuity of care reflected in higher utilization of services. Case management services are critical in connecting older adults with HIV to needed services, particularly those services that are not AIDS service organization-based but, rather, community based and largely government funded (see Table 5). The use of case management was more likely for those connected to the entitlement system (i.e., Medicaid-enrolled), as well as for those expressing greater need for services in the previous year (see Table 4). As was the case for the use of other services, there was no significant effect due to sexual identity/gender on the use of case management in bivariate and multivariate analyses.

With regard to service need variables tested in our Andersen Model (Andersen, 1968, 1995) regressions, both level of depressive symptoms and self-reported service needs in the previous year were significant covariates of service utilization. Depression was related to greater service use overall, the use of government offices/agencies and, not surprisingly, health and long-term care services. Expressed need for services was significantly related to utilization overall, and within every domain with the exception of government agencies and offices. Thus, service use in the population aging with HIV appears to be driven by need factors and enabling factors that facilitate access to services. These findings parallel what has been reported about service utilization among older adults in general—namely, that predisposing factors play a small role when enabling factors such as connections to the entitlement system and need for services are considered (Cantor & Brennan, 1993, 2000). Previous research has found that PLWHA have high levels of service needs, and many unmet needs for services including needed assistance from governmental authorities, community agencies, religious institutions, and help in obtaining entitlements. For example, Kupprat,

Dayton, Guschlbauer, and Halkitis (2009) in a chart review of HIV-positive women found that less than one-half had accessed mental health and substance use treatment, despite very high rates of mental illness and substance use, suggesting there is an unmet need for these services. Furthermore, there is evidence that PLWHA who are not in medical care have greater unmet needs compared to their peers who are not receiving such care (Tobias et al., 2007).

It is important to underscore that service utilization among older adults with HIV is significantly higher when compared to non-infected peers. If we consider only the subset of 15 non-HIV related services examined in Cantor and Brennan's (1993, 2000) work on service utilization among older adults (i.e., Social Security, Medicaid, Medicare, Human Resources Administration, homecare, visiting nurse, nursing home, VA/VA hospital, emergency room, inpatient hospital, senior center, Department for the Aging, Housing Authority, police, and clergy), we find that this sample of OPLWHA are using 3.6 services, on average, which is significantly greater than the 1.0 services used among community-dwelling older adults 65 and older, $t(1,888) = 21.16$, $p < .001$. This is likely a function of a number of factors, including greater service needs driven by a high level of comorbid physical and mental health challenges, and a lack of informal social resources. This intense reliance on formal support services is predicted by Cantor's Hierarchical Compensatory Theory (Cantor & Mayer, 1978), which suggests that when informal supports are not available the older adult increasingly relies on formal services for support.

Policy and Program Implications

Case management and service utilization. Case management emerged as a significant enabling factor for virtually all types of service utilization among OPLWHA in this study. It has been identified as an important service use covariate in other studies of people living with HIV (Anthony et al., 2007; W. E. Cunningham et al., 2008; London et al., 1998). Among older adults receiving formal services, case management has been associated with lower depression, particularly in older adults without informal supports (Muramatsu, Yin, & Hedeker, 2010). Our finding that Medicaid enrollment significantly increased the odds of using case management is congruent with other research that points to greater utilization of this service among those who are economically disadvantaged (Basta et al., 2008; C. O. Cunningham, Sanchez, Li, Heller, & Sohler, 2008). Unfortunately, in the current reduction of services to PLWHA arising from funding cuts from the federal, state, and local governments, there have been efforts to constrict access to case management services in this population (Thorpe, 2011). Our findings, as well of those of Ohl et al. (2008), suggest that case management is an important point of entry to the service system. Access to this service should be protected and facilitated to meet the high level of need among OPLWHA.

Mainstreaming the older adult with HIV. The significant utilization of non-HIV-related services reported in this article reinforces the policy conclusions of the ROAH study (Brennan et al., 2009). That large scale study of 1000 OPLWHA in New York City concluded that the support needs of this population can best be addressed by their being mainstreamed into the existing service structure of community-based organizations that provide services to older adults. Economically and structurally, the network of HIV providers is unlikely to have the capacity and expertise to provide all the services needed by an aging HIV population. Concomitantly, the needs of this aging population are in line with the existing services available from senior service providers. Such mainstreaming efforts will also begin to ameliorate the prevalent levels of stigma and reduce endemic social isolation that these older adults experience (Brennan & Karpiak, 2009; Cantor et al., 2009).

Supporting HIV/AIDS treatment services. Service utilization findings from this study underscore the critical need for supportive services for people living with HIV/AIDS. Since the financial and economic crisis of 2008 evolved into a fiscal crisis for state and local governments, funding for HIV services that complement medical care has decreased and failed to keep pace with the a growing and aging HIV population. The 111th Congress has also threatened to cut funding for HIV care. Given the expanded HIV testing campaigns supported by the CDC to find the estimated one-in-five people living with HIV who are unaware of their status, and the estimated 56,000 Americans newly diagnosed each year, it is critical that funding for the Ryan White Care Act, the AIDS Drug Assistance Program, and other programs be maintained at sufficient levels. It is also essential to continue to fund these programs in order to improve treatment outcomes, a key goal of the President's National HIV/AIDS Strategy.

Mental health and substance use issues: Stigma and social isolation. The high rates of depressive symptomatology found in the sample, with more than one-half moderately or severely depressed, underscore the critical role of mental health services, and the nexus between mental and physical health. More important, depression was significantly related to higher levels of service utilization. Effective mental health treatment, which could alleviate depression and potentially reduce service demand, must be affordable and culturally competent to serve OPLWHA and older GLBT adults. The high rate of depression in a population that is receiving intensive medical care and community-based services is troubling and suggest the need for more research to determine the etiology of depression in this group, as well as a review of policies and standards of mental health care to better address this problem. Of course, there is a significant overlap between mental health and substance use issues. Nearly 40% of the heterosexual respondents, 21% of bisexual men, and 15% of homosexual men in the sample reported using substance use treatment and recovery services. Furthermore, although providing mental health services that are accessible to OPLWHA is important, we should also address structural correlates of depression, including stigma and social isolation (Grov, Golub, Parsons, Brennan, & Karpiak, 2010), and seek to ameliorate and eliminate them. This will require helping OPLWHAs address HIV disclosure issues, which serve to reinforce their self-imposed isolation (Emlet, 2006).

The need for socialization. The highest stated unmet need of this study population for all four groups was socialization. The expression of this need reinforces the observed fragility and inadequacy of this population's social networks (Cantor et al., 2009; Shippy & Karpiak, 2005b). Our current findings indicate that the needs of this population are large and are being met through accessing multiple formal services. But, the level of need for these formal services would likely be reduced if this population were better able to socialize and create connections—namely, social networks, from which informal support is derived. In addition, unpaid caregivers are typically drawn from the informal social network, so enhancing these informal resources will assist OPLWHA to meet their current and future caregiving needs. Informal caregiving had an annual value of approximately $450 billion in the United States in 2009 (AARP Public Policy Institute, 2011). Thus, findings from this study support the conclusion that improving socialization opportunities for OPLWHA could be a worthwhile investment, resulting in a significant reduction in the use, and subsequent cost, of formal services. In addition, AIDS service organizations and GLBT community centers should educate people living with HIV and AIDS about resources available under the National Family Caregiver Support Program, which uses an inclusive definition of the term "caregiver" to encompass same-sex partners and close friends.

An older population of "greatest social need." Findings that more than one-half of these GMHC clients age 50 years and older had received an AIDS diagnosis and had, on average, 3.4 comorbid conditions in addition to HIV defines these OPLWHA as a vulnerable population with specific health care needs. The *Older Americans Act* (OAA; National Council on Aging, 2013), which funds more than $2 billion per year in senior services, should be amended to list older adults living with HIV, as well as older GLBT adults in general, as among the populations who are aging in the United States with "greatest social need." Their vulnerability is exacerbated due to HIV stigma, as well as anti-gay bias in senior settings among peers and staff (Behney, 1994; Crisp, 2006; Emlet, 2006, 2007; Knochel, Croghan, Moone, & Quam, 2010). Designating OPLWHA and GLBT older adults as populations of "greatest social need" would direct state and regional aging agencies to explicitly incorporate the unique needs of these populations into their 5-year aging plans. OAA-funded agencies should at a minimum promote cultural competency training for senior service providers, challenge stigma among staff and peers in senior settings, and promote HIV prevention among all older adults who are at-risk.

Strengths and Limitations

This study had a number of strengths, including having a unique and comprehensive data set on older adults with HIV data to compare heterosexual, homosexual, and bisexual groups, and a conceptually based multivariate analysis based on the Andersen Model (Andersen, 1968, 1995). However, there are limitations to the findings. The sample of adults 50 years and older was drawn from a single AIDS service organization in New York City, and due to the lack of an established sample frame for OPLWHA, it is unclear if these findings would generalize to clients from other AIDS service organizations in other cities. In addition, New York City and State have a particularly rich service environment compared to many other areas of the country, which may affect levels of utilization, as well as covariates of service use. Due to sample limitations, we were unable to examine the experience of older lesbian/bisexual women or transgender individuals with HIV and, therefore, cannot confidently generalize these findings to these groups.

CONCLUSION

We recently marked the 30th anniversary of the HIV/AIDS epidemic. At the end of the third decade, we see the results of effective antiretroviral therapies. These drugs have transformed HIV/AIDS from a rapidly progressing terminal disease to a chronic illness. The success of treatments has given a longer life span to those who would otherwise have died. This is a resilient population that is confronting considerable challenges that cannot be ignored if they are to age successfully. Over two-thirds live alone, and many are isolated from friends and families due to the persistent toxic effects of AIDS-related stigma (Emlet, 2007). Many are afraid to tell others that they have HIV disease, fearing both rejection and even violence (Brennan & Karpiak, 2009; Emlet 2006). As a consequence most have fragile social networks that are unable to support them as they age (Shippy & Karpiak 2005a, 2005b). Ostracized, they withdraw, exacerbating high rates of depressive symptoms, which are five times higher when compared to their peers who are not living with HIV. Without the social supports from which care and assistance can be obtained, this aging population will be relegated to costly home health care services and long-term care facilities in the coming decades. Will an already overburdened health and social care system be able to meet their increased needs? Funding streams to AIDS service organizations must reflect the burden of disease seen among those aging with HIV. These challenges also require testing innovative approaches that will end the stigma-driven social isolation that too many of these individuals endure, and also provide the social supports, both formal and informal, that they will need in the coming decades.

REFERENCES

AARP Public Policy Institute. (2011). *Valuing the invaluable: 2011 update— The growing contributions and costs of family caregiving.* Washington, DC: Author. Retrieved from http://www.aarp.org/relationships/caregiving/info-07-2011/valuing-the-invaluable.html

Andersen, E. M., Malmgren, J. A., Carter, W. B., & Patrick, D. L. (1994). Screening for depression in well older adults: Evaluation of a short form of the CES–D (Center for Epidemiological Studies Depression Scale). *American Journal of Preventive Medicine, 10*(2), 77–84.

Andersen, R. M. (1968). *Behavioral model of families' use of health services* (Research Series No. 25). Chicago, IL: University of Chicago, Center for Health Administration Studies.

Andersen, R. M. (1995). Revisiting the behavioral model and access to medical care: Does it matter? *Journal of Health and Social Behavior, 36*(1), 1–10.

Anthony, M. N., Gardner, L., Marks, G., Anderson-Mahoney, P., Metsch, L. R., Valverde, E. E., Loughlin, A. M. (2007). Factors associated with use of HIV primary care among persons recently diagnosed with HIV: Examination of variables from the behavioral model of health-care utilization. *AIDS Care, 19*, 195–202.

Basta, T., Shacham, E., & Reece, M. (2008). Psychological distress and engagement in HIV-related services among individuals seeking mental health care. *AIDS Care, 20*, 969–976.

Behney, R. (1994). The Aging Network's response to gay and lesbian issues. *Outword: Newsletter of the Lesbian and Gay Aging Issues Networks, 1*(2), 2. San Francisco, CA: Lesbian and Gay Aging Issues Network of the American Society on Aging.

Bell, S. A., Bern-Klug, M., Kramer, K. W., & Saunders, J. B. (2010). Most nursing home social service directors lack training in working with lesbian, gay and bisexual residents. *Social Work in Health Care, 49*, 814–831.

Bettencourt, T., Hodgins, A., Huba, G. J., & Pickett, G. (1998). Bay area young positives: A model of a youth-based approach to HIV/AIDS services. *Journal of Adolescent Health, 23*(Suppl. 2), 28–36.

Bjerk, S. (2011, May 9). *Mayor Bloomberg's executive budget tramples on basic human rights* [Web log post]. Retrieved from http://www.housingworks.org/blogs/detail/mayor-bloombergs-executive-budget-tramples-on-basic-human-rights/

Brennan, M., & Karpiak, S. E. (2009). HIV stigma and disclosure of serostatus. In M. Brennan, S. E. Karpiak, R. A. Shippy, & M. H. Cantor (Eds.), *Research on Older Adults with HIV: An in-depth examination of an emerging population* (pp. 51–60). New York, NY: Nova Science.

Brennan, M., Karpiak, S. E., Shippy, R. A., & Cantor, M. H. (Eds.). (2009). *Older adults with HIV: An in-depth examination of an emerging population*. New York, NY: Nova Science.

Brennan, M., Strauss, S. M., & Karpiak, S. E. (2010). Religious congregations and the growing needs of older adults with HIV. *Journal of Religion, Spirituality, and Aging, 22*, 307–328.

Brotman, S., Ryan, B., & Cormier, R. (2003). The health and service needs of gay and lesbian elders and their families in Canada. *Gerontologist, 43*, 192–202.

Burnam, M. A., Bing, E. G., Morton, S. C., Sherbourne, C., Feishman, J. A., London, A. S., Shapiro, M. F. (2001). Use of mental health and substance abuse treatment services among adults with HIV in the United States. *Archives of General Psychiatry, 58*, 729–744.

Cantor, M. H., & Brennan, M. (1993). *Family and community support systems of older New Yorkers. Growing older in New York City in the 1990s: A study of changing lifestyles, quality of life, and quality of care, Vol. V*. New York, NY: New York Center for Policy on Aging, New York Community Trust.

Cantor, M. H., & Brennan, M. (2000). *Social care of the elderly: The effects of ethnicity, class, and culture*. New York, NY: Springer.

Cantor, M. H., Brennan, M., & Karpiak, S. E. (2009). The social support networks of older people with HIV. In M. Brennan, S. E. Karpiak, R. A. Shippy, & M. H. Cantor (Eds.), *Research on Older Adults with HIV: An in-depth examination of an emerging population* (pp. 61–74). New York, NY: Nova Science.

Cantor, M. H., Brennan, M., & Shippy, R. A. (2004). *Caregiving among older lesbian, gay, bisexual, and transgender New Yorkers. Final report*. Washington, DC: National Gay and Lesbian Task Force Policy Institute.

Cantor, M. H., & Mayer, M. (1978). Factors in differential utilization of services by urban elderly. *Journal of Gerontological Social Work, 1*(1), 47–61.

Centers for Disease Control and Prevention. (2008). *HIV/AIDS among persons 50 and older*. Atlanta, GA: Author. Retrieved from http://www.cdc.gov/hiv/topics/over50/resources/factsheets/pdf/over50.pdf

Crisp, C. (2006). The Gay Affirmative Practice scale (GAP): A new measure for assessing cultural competence with gay and lesbian clients. *Social Work, 51*, 115–126.

Cunningham, C. O., Sanchez, J., Li, X., Heller D., & Sohler, N. I. (2008). Medical and support service utilization in a medical program targeting marginalized HIV-infected individuals. *Journal of Health Care for the Poor and Underserved, 19*, 981–990.

Cunningham, W. E., Wong, M., & Hays, R. D. (2008). Case management and health-related quality of life outcomes in a national sample of persons with HIV/AIDS. *Journal of the National Medical Association, 100*, 840–847.

Effros, R., Fletcher, C., Gebo, K., Halter, J. B., Hazzard, W., Horne, F., . . . High, K. P., (2008). Workshop on HIV infection and aging: What is known and future research directions. *Clinical Infectious Diseases, 47*, 542–553.

Emlet, C. (2006). "You're awfully old to have this disease": Experiences of stigma and ageism in adults 50 years and older living with HIV/AIDS. *Gerontologist, 46*, 781–790.

Emlet, C. (2007). Experiences of stigma in older adults living with HIV/AIDS: A mixed-method analysis. *AIDS Patient Care and STDs, 21,* 740–752.

Fritsch, T. (2005). HIV/AIDS and the older adult: An exploratory study of the age-related differences in access to medical and social services. *Journal of Applied Gerontology, 24*(1), 35–54.

Grov, C., Golub, S. A., Parsons, J. T., Brennan, M., & Karpiak, S. E. (2010). Loneliness and HIV-related stigma explain depression among older HIV-positive adults. *AIDS Care, 22,* 630–639.

Havlik, R. J. (2009). Health status, comorbidities, and health-related quality of life. In M. Brennan, S. E. Karpiak, R. A. Shippy, & M. H. Cantor (Eds.), *Research on Older Adults with HIV: An in-depth examination of an emerging population* (pp. 13–25). New York, NY: Nova Science.

Havlik, R. J., Brennan, M., & Karpiak, S. E. (2011). Comorbidities and depression in older adults with HIV. *Sexual Health, 8,* 551–559. doi:10.1071/SH11017

Hughes, M. (2007). Older lesbians and gays accessing health and aged-care services. *Australian Social Work, 60,* 197–209.

Institute of Medicine. (2011). *The health of lesbian, gay, bisexual and transgender people: Building a foundation for better understanding.* Washington, DC: National Academies Press.

Karpiak, S. E., & Brennan, M. (2009). The emerging population of older adults with HIV and introduction to the ROAH study. In M. Brennan, S. E. Karpiak, R. A. Shippy, & M. H. Cantor (Eds.), *Older adults with HIV: An in-depth examination of an emerging population* (pp. 1–12). New York, NY: Nova Science.

Knochel, K. A., Croghan, C., Moone, R., & Quam, J. (2010). *Ready to serve? Pfund Foundation report on the aging network and lesbian, gay, bisexual and transgender older adults.* Minneapolis, MN: Pfund and the College of Education and Human Development, University of Minnesota. Retrieved from http://www.pfundonline.org/pdf/Ready_to_Serve_PFundReport.pdf

Kupprat, S. A., Dayton, A., Guschlbauer, A., & Halkitis, P. N. (2009). Case manager-reported utilization of support group, substance use and mental health services among HIV-positive women in New York City. *AIDS Care, 21,* 874–880.

London, A. S., Fleishman, J. A., Goldman, D. P., McCaffrey, D. F., Bozzette, S. A., Shapiro, M. F., & Liebowitz, A. A. (2001). Use of unpaid and paid home care services among people with HIV infection in the USA. *AIDS Care, 13,* 99–121.

London, A. S., LeBlanc, A. J., & Aneshensel, C. S. (1998). The integration of informal care, case management and community-based services for persons with HIV. *AIDS Care, 10,* 481–503.

Masini, B. E., & Barrett, H. A. (2008). Social support as a predictor of psychological and physical well-being and lifestyle in lesbian, gay, and bisexual adults aged 50 and over. *Journal of Gay and Lesbian Social Services,* 20(1/2), 91–110.

Muramatsu, N., Yin, H., & Hedeker, D. (2010). Functional declines, social support, and mental health in the elderly: Does living in a state supportive of home and community-based services make a difference? *Social Science and Medicine, 70,* 1050–1058.

National Council on Aging. (2013). *Older Americans Act reauthorization.* Retrieved November 4, 2013 from: http://www.ncoa.org/public-policy-action/older-americans-act/

Ohl, M. E., Landon, B. E., Clearly, P. D., & LeMaster, J. (2008). Medical clinical characteristics and access to behavioral health services for persons with HIV. *Psychiatric Services*, *59*, 400–407.

Penniman, T. V., Taylor, S. L., Bird, C. E., Beckman, R., Collins, R. L., & Cunningham, W. (2007). The associations of gender, sexual identity and competing needs with healthcare utilization among people with HIV/AIDS. *Journal of the National Medical Association*, *99*, 419–427.

Radloff, L. S. (1977). The CES–D Scale: A self report depression scale for research in the general population. *Applied Psychological Measurement*, *1*, 385–401.

Sheehan, N. W., Wilson, R., & Marella, L. M. (1988). The role of church in providing services for the aging. *Journal of Applied Gerontology*, *7*, 231–241.

Shippy, R. A., Cantor, M. H., & Brennan, M. (2004). Social networks of aging gay men. *Journal of Men's Studies*, *13*(1), 107–120.

Shippy, R. A., & Karpiak, S. E. (2005a). The aging HIV/AIDS population: Fragile social networks. *Aging & Mental Health*, *9*, 246–254.

Shippy, R. A., & Karpiak, S. E. (2005b). Perceptions of support among older adults with HIV. *Research on Aging*, *27*, 290–306.

Smith, L. A., McCaslin, R., Chang, J., Martinez, P., & McGrew, P. (2010). Assessing the needs of older gay, lesbian, bisexual and transgender people: A service-learning and agency partnership approach. *Journal of Gerontological Social Work*, *53*, 387–401.

Tan, P. P. (2005). The importance of spirituality among gay and lesbian individuals. *Journal of Homosexuality*, *49*(2), 135–144.

Tirrito, T., & Choi, G. (2005). Faith organizations and ethnically diverse elders: A community-action model. *Journal of Religious Gerontology*, 16(1/2), 123–142.

Tjepkema, M. (2008). Health care use among gay, lesbian and bisexual Canadians. *Health Reports*, *19*(1), 53–64.

Tobias, C. R., Cunningham, W., Cabral, H. D., Cunningham, C. O., Eldred, L., Naar-King, S., Drainoni, M. L. (2007). Living with HIV but without medical care: Barriers to engagement. *AIDS Patient Care and STDs*, *21*, 426–434.

Walensky, R. P., Paltiel, A. D., Losina, E., Mercincavage, L. M., Schackman, B. R., Sax, P. E., Freedberg, K. A. (2006). The survival benefits of AIDS treatment in the United States. *Journal of Infectious Diseases*, *194*, 11–19.

Do LGBT Aging Trainings Effectuate Positive Change in Mainstream Elder Service Providers?

KRISTEN E. PORTER, MS, MAc

Department of Gerontology, John E. McCormack School of Policy & Global Studies,
University of Massachusetts, Boston, Massachusetts, USA

LISA KRINSKY, MSW, LICSW

The LGBT Aging Project, The Fenway Institute, Fenway Health, Boston, Massachusetts, USA

This study aims to provide empirical evidence regarding whether attitudes, beliefs, and intentions of elder-service providers can be positively affected as a result of attending cultural competency training on the unique challenges of sexual and gender minorities. Stigmatization throughout the lifespan may have a causal influence on barriers to care, social isolation, and concomitant health disparities. Data were collected for this study at 4 Massachusetts training events to pilot a cultural competency workshop on lesbian, gay, bisexual, and transgender (LGBT) aging for mainstream elder service providers. This quasi-experimental study included the analysis of pre- and posttest surveys completed by the service-provider attendees (N = 76). The analytic strategy included descriptive statistics, paired t tests, chi-square analyses, and repeated measures analyses of variance. Findings revealed statistically significant improvement in numerous aspects of providers' knowledge, attitudes, and behavioral intentions subsequent to the training sessions. These included (p = .000) awareness of LGBT resources, policy disparities, spousal benefits for same-sex couples, and the intention to challenge homophobic remarks. This study concludes that mainstream elder-service provider training on LGBT aging issues results in positive change. Recommendations include

The authors would like to acknowledge the work of John Snow Inc. Research and Training Institute, especially Dianne Perlmutter and Jodi Sperber; Jeff Burr, PhD for guidance; and Brian de Vries, PhD for his vision and technical assistance.

long-term follow up of participants, the inception of agency-level surveys to appraise institutional culture change, and increased curriculum on transgender older adults.

In the United States, demographers expect the population of lesbian, gay, bisexual, and transgender (LGBT) older adults, currently estimated at around two million people, to double by 2030 (Fredriksen-Goldsen et al., 2011). The U.S. Administration on Aging, Department of Health and Human Services acknowledges that elder-care institutions and agencies may lack sensitivity toward the unique needs and circumstances of the LGBT aging population, resulting in discrimination against this minority population across the range of services (Administration on Aging [AOA], 2010; John Snow Inc. [JSI], 2003). The future growth of this population, along with the history of discrimination against them, provides a timely opportunity for elder service providers to engage in evidence-based strategies to develop LGBT cultural competence.

LGBT older adults, as a consequence of their sexual minority status, experience financial, social and economic discrimination; physical and mental abuse; and lack of access to quality, culturally sensitive health care (Connolly, 1996; Grant, Koskovich, Frazer, & Bjerk, 2010; Institute of Medicine [IOM], 2011; MetLife, 2010; Turner, Wilson, & Shirah, 2006). This group may also rely upon aging services, home care, and institutionalized care in elevated degrees compared to their heterosexual counterparts due in part to demographic and policy factors. These factors include the lack of transferrable spousal benefits through Social Security and the Veteran's Administration; a greater percentage living alone (33% of LGBTs compared to 18% of heterosexuals; MetLife, 2010); and the majority do not have children to provide familial caregiving (AOA, 2010; Cahill & South, 2002; Grant et al., 2010; Stein, Beckerman, & Sherman, 2010).

Health disparities for LGBT older adults are well documented across multiple dimensions (IOM, 2011; Mayer et al., 2008). Cultural sensitivity training is a strategic approach to mitigate health disparities by developing provider proficiency in understanding the unique needs of diverse cultural groups; the LGBT community is now recognized as one such minority group (AOA, 2010, Grant et al., 2010; Turner et al., 2006; Van Den Bergh & Crisp, 2004). Providing LGBT cultural competency training is a micro-level intervention recommended to service providers of older adults, however, there has been little evaluation of its efficacy (Grant et al., 2010).

PURPOSE OF THIS STUDY

This study aims to provide empirical evidence regarding whether attitudes, beliefs, and intentions of elder-service staff can be positively affected as a result of attending cultural competency training on the unique challenges and needs of LGBT older adults. This study included a pre- and posttest evaluation of a 5-hr pilot training workshop on LGBT aging developed for service providers of older adults. This training program was created by members of the elder service community with funding from The Gill Foundation. This provides a formal evaluation of this training program. The specific goal of the study was to measure changes in knowledge, attitudes and behavioral intentions as a result of participation in the trainings.

LITERATURE REVIEW

Understanding a Lifetime of Stigma

The IOM's (2011) health report reveals that most LGBT older adults have been stigmatized and marginalized throughout the lifespan, including by the federal government, the military, medical providers, and other mainstream agencies. Stigmatization of LGBT people is rooted in the constructs of heterosexism and homophobia, and is understood to include labeling, stereotyping, status loss, and discrimination (Link & Phelan, 2001). Homophobia, the fear and hatred of those perceived to be gay, and heterosexism, the belief in heterosexual superiority, together, perpetuate a system of institutionalized stigma that pervades elder care service systems (Crisp, 2006; Grant et al., 2010; Morrow, 2001). Long-term care settings, senior centers, elder home care agencies, and other health and social service providers have discriminated against LGBT older adults based upon sexual orientation by denying care or providing care that was inferior or neglectful (AOA, 2010; Johnson, Jackson, Arnette, & Koffman, 2005; JSI, 2003; National Senior Citizens Law Center, 2011). For example, the prevailing assumption by service providers is that all older adults are heterosexual, also known as heteronormativism (AOA, 2010; Crisp, 2006; Turner et al., 2006); this institutionalized heterosexism results in a narrow understanding of the lives, needs, and priorities of LGBT older adults. In addition, this institutionalized heterosexism serves as a barrier to care for LGBT older adults, leaving this marginalized minority population even more vulnerable as they age.

As a result of enacted, felt, or internalized stigma, LGBT older adults often avoid using traditional elder services due to the lack of specific LGBT programming, feeling unwelcomed, or the assumption that staff may not be sensitive to their needs (Butler, 2004; IOM, 2011). The MetLife Mature Market Institute (2010) study found that 10% of LGBT older adults fear they will encounter discrimination because of their sexual identity and 45% expressed some concern about whether they would be treated with respect by health professionals. Older generations, many already residing in residential facilities, voice strong fear of mistreatment and neglect by care providers (Stein et al., 2010). A New York study revealed that for LGBT older adults age 60 to 84, 38% do not disclose their sexual orientation to their medical providers, 30% had a poor experience when doing so, and 13% chose not to seek medical care due to fear of the provider's reaction to their sexual orientation (Stein et al., 2010). Thus, both the perceived fear of stigma, and past experience of discrimination, contributes to barriers accessing care that can negatively impact the health and well-being of LGBT older adults. This is the sort of interaction-behavior relationship described by Meyer (2003) in the *minority stress* model. In this model, a person who experiences social stigma due to his or her minority status develops an internal landscape of additive stress, cumulating in negative health consequences. The minority stress that is produced contributes to concealment of identity by LGBT older adults along with underutilization of mainstream support services.

These beliefs and fears are well justified as the research literature demonstrates widespread anti-gay bias among service providers, including discrimination, refusal to touch, physical and verbal abuse, inappropriate curiosity, denial of care, and breach of confidentiality (Brotman, Cormier, & Ryan, 2001; Fairchild, Carrino, & Ramirez, 1996; Grant et al., 2010; JSI, 2003; O'Hanlan, Cabaj, Schatz, Lock, & Nemrow, 1997). Fredriksen-Goldsen et al. (2011) found that more than 13% of LGBT older adults "report being denied or provided inferior healthcare because they are LGBT, and 4% have experienced this three or more times in their life" (p. 31). Stein et al.'s (2010) study showed that 83% of LGBT elders experienced stigma directly from health care providers. Anti-gay bias was directly witnessed in half of medical providers as reported by medical students (O'Hanlan et al., 1997). A study of 29 nursing homes revealed that more than half of the direct-care staff was "condemning" or "intolerant" of homosexuality (Fairchild et al., 1996, p. 161). Likewise, a New York Area Agencies on Aging (AAA) study revealed 96% of the 29 agencies surveyed had no programming for LGBT elders, and the majority of senior centers in those areas stated they would not be welcoming of openly gay elders (Fairchild et al., 1996). Not surprising, only 19% of LGBT elders interviewed in those covered areas belonged to the local senior center (Grant et al., 2010).

As a result of this stigma, and their own experiences, LGBT older adults often live with a chronic fear of discrimination (IOM, 2011). There is now strong evidence linking the stigmatization of LGBT older adults with abuse; for example, 68% of older LGBT adults have been verbally assaulted and 19% have been physically assaulted (Fredriksen-Goldsen et al., 2011). LGBT elder abuse is often unreported due to fear that doing so may result in caregiver threats to disclose the elder's sexual orientation or gender identity as a reporting consequence (Grant et al., 2010). In the cases documented, perpetrators allude to the following explanations for their abusive behavior: fear of AIDS transmission, stigmatizing religious beliefs (Shankle, Maxwell,

Katzman, & Landers, 2003), and overall negative attitudes toward same-sex sexual activity (Hinrichs & Vacha-Haase, 2010). Among more than half of LGBT elders fearing abuse (National Senior Citizens Law Center, 2011; Stein et al., 2010), at least one-third anticipate they will not disclose their sexual orientation to elder service staff as a defensive strategy (Johnson et al., 2005). The statistics are even more alarming for LGBT residents of long term care facilities; only 22% feel they can be candid about their sexual orientation or gender identity to facility staff and 43% reported abuse as a result of revealing their sexual orientation or gender identity (National Senior Citizens Law Center, 2011). The research literature shows there is clearly a need for education and intervention to address these problems.

LGBT CULTURAL COMPETENCY TRAINING

Training agency staff and providers on the unique needs and challenges of LGBT older adults provides a vehicle to attenuate stigma, with the goal of diminishing or eliminating the discrimination noted earlier (AOA, 2010; Grant et al., 2010; Turner et al., 2006). Although an individual or agency cannot develop competence in another culture per say, *cultural competency* is the adopted terminology defined as "a set of skills that allows providers to give culturally appropriate high-quality care to individuals of cultures different from their own" (IOM, 2011, p. 65). We use the terms *competency, sensitivity,* and *awareness* interchangeably to represent the individual or agency development of attitudes, skills, and practices that reflect the acknowledgment of unique characteristics and experiences for identified populations and communities. Although many elder service agencies provide in-service trainings for staff, LGBT aging training is not commonly offered. A recently published national study surveyed over 1,000 nursing home directors and reported that 75% had less than 1 hr of training over the past 5 years on homophobia, heterosexism, and LGBT awareness (Bell, Bern-Klug, Kramer, & Saunders, 2010).

Few published reports evaluate the benefits of LGBT cultural competency training; however, medical research associates culturally sensitive care with improved health outcomes for patients (Crandall, George, Marion, & Davis, 2003). A 2000 Massachusetts study of 324 health care providers who attended a LGBT health access training reported favorable change in provider attitudes toward LGBT persons, however, the results were not statistically significant (Clark, Landers, Linde, & Sperber, 2001). A 2004 study of 91 medical students trained in cultural competence (not a training specific to the LGBT population) showed significant improvement from pre-to post-training using the Health Beliefs Attitudes Survey (Crosson, Deng, Brazeau, Boyd, & Soto-Greene, 2004). Thus, anecdotal evidence suggests that LGBT cultural competency training for elder service providers could increase the professional capacity of staff, encourage dialogue about sexuality in general, and help create more welcoming environments for LGBT older adults. This study aims to document if empirical evidence exists to support these claims.

LGBT OLDER ADULTS OF MASSACHUSETTS: FOCUS ON HOME CARE STUDY

This study evaluates a Massachusetts training program that was developed by LGBT-identified providers working in the elder service profession. The curriculum developers' knowledge and experience in both the aging profession and the LGBT community enhanced the relevance of the content; ensuring that the curriculum addressed the most significant issues in both fields. The LGBT Aging Project adopted this curriculum to augment mainstream elder services professional capacity to provide dignified and respectful care to LGBT older adults. The LGBT community's initiative to bring cultural awareness to mainstream aging was in keeping with the historical precedent of taking care of one's own, a philosophically rooted response to crisis and adaptation of self-efficacy that developed during the HIV/AIDS epidemic (Fredriksen-Goldsen et al., 2011; IOM, 2011).

METHOD

Data Source

Data were collected at four training events held in Eastern Massachusetts in 2003 to pilot a cultural competency workshop on LGBT aging for mainstream elder service providers. The study, funded by the Medical Foundation/Farnsworth Trust, was a partnership between the JSI and the Massachusetts LGBT Aging Project. The study included the analysis of pre- and posttest surveys completed by the service-provider attendees who participated in the LGBT cultural competency trainings and was approved by the institutional review board at the University of Massachusetts, Boston.

Study Sample

In this quasi-experimental study, individuals were the unit of analysis, with elder-service providers as the target population. The sample for this analysis included a range of personnel, all of whom were employed at four separate Area Agencies on Aging (AAAs). The AAAs provide referrals, case management, adult protective services and other community based services for older adults. Participants were recruited through flyers posted at the AAA locations and advertisements in agency newsletters ($N = 76$). Participants received no incentives and participation was voluntary.

Procedures

The training facilitator, a member of the LGBT Aging Project, conducted the 5-hr workshop at each of the four training sites. The learning objectives in the curriculum included (a) addressing the myths and realities of LGBT aging, (b) exploring prejudice and identifying barriers to providing quality services for LGBT older adults, and (c) developing strategies for improving access and enhancing knowledge about public policies of importance to LGBT older adults. A pretest was administered as participants arrived at the training session; a posttest was administered at the end of the training session with no control group. Both surveys were identical tools asking an array of 32 questions to ascertain demographics, knowledge, attitudes, and behavioral intentions. The pre- and posttest took approximately 15 min each to complete and were anonymous. To ensure anonymity, each participant created a unique respondent code so that pre- and posttests could be compared. The completed surveys, sealed in an unidentified envelope, were collected by the facilitator and submitted to JSI. To be considered complete, both a pre- and a posttest had to be submitted by each participant, otherwise the data were discarded. Seventy-six participants submitted complete data.

Measures

The pre- and posttest questionnaire comprised several sections. Section A contained 15 five-point Likert scale questions (*strongly agree* to *strongly disagree*) pertaining to respondent comfort level, awareness and attitudes such as comfort in being in the home of an LGBT person, awareness of resources for LGBT elders and federal policy disparities, and attitudes about spousal benefits. Examples of these questions include, "I am/would be comfortable providing services to an openly gay, lesbian, or bisexual elder," "I am/would be comfortable providing services to an openly transgender elder," "Each of us contributes to the homophobia in our society," "My agency should provide services specifically targeted to LGBT elders," "Intake forms should give a person the opportunity to disclose their sexual orientation and gender identity," and "I am aware of policy disparities that affect LGBT elders."

Section B included seven dichotomous questions (true or false) assessing knowledge about federal policies and disparities. Examples of these questions include, "Life partners of LGBT persons are entitled to the same social security benefits as spouses," "LGBT elders have an increased risk of untreated serious illnesses," "Homosexuality is a diagnosis of mental disorder in the mental health community's *Diagnostic and Statistical Manual*," and "Federal housing programs mandate non-discrimination based upon sexual orientation."

Section C contained 4 five-point Likert scale questions (*never* to *always*) and one dichotomous question (yes or no) assessing behaviors. These questions asked, "I think I can tell whether an elder is heterosexual or homosexual," "When describing romantic relationships, I use inclusive words (e.g., partner, significant other), in addition to words like girlfriend, boyfriend, husband, and wife," "When I hear homophobic or transphobic jokes or comments, I am willing to challenge those who make them," "I assume that the elders I serve are heterosexual," and "I currently have objects in my office that create a welcoming environment for gay, lesbian, bisexual, and transgender elders." For analysis purposes, this last yes/no question is reported as part of section B along with the other dichotomous questions.

Section D asked demographic questions. Gender asked, "My sex/gender is," and was measured as female = 1, male = 2, male-to-female transgender = 3, and female-to-male transgender = 4. Race/ethnicity asked, "My race/ethnicity is (check all that apply)," and was measured by 10 answer categories including "other." Sexual orientation asked, "My sexual orientation is," and was measured by bisexual = 1, gay/lesbian = 2, heterosexual = 3, and other = 4. To compare differences based on sexual orientation, the variable was recoded to a dichotomous variable, with heterosexual = 0 and non-heterosexuals = 1. Finally, LGBT training experience was measured by instructing respondents to "fill out before training only: have you previously participated in training on gay, lesbian, bisexual, and transgender issues," with yes = 1 and no = 0. In addition, the survey asked "job class (circle one)" with response categories of administrative support, direct services, and manager/supervisor.

Analytic Strategy

This data analysis included several steps. All data were coded and checked for quality control. Descriptive statistics were provided for the sociodemographic variables. Paired t tests and chi-square analyses were used to measure statistical significance of the pre- and posttest comparisons. Various supplemental analyses were run to assess if the t test results were driven by group differences between providers identifying as heterosexual compared to those identifying as LGBT. These included running an additional series of t test analyses or analyses of variance (ANOVAs), where appropriate, comparing heterosexual participants with LGBT participants on the continuous measures; chi-square analyses were conducted on the dichotomous measures. Results are discussed in the next section. Statistical Package for the Social Sciences software Version 19 (SPSS, Inc., Chicago, IL) was used.

RESULTS

Descriptive Statistics

The descriptive statistics in Table 1 showed that of the 76 service providers that participated, 69 identified as female, 6 identified as men and one identified as female to male transgender. The providers were predominately

TABLE 1 Sociodemographic Sample Characteristics of Study Participants in Lesbian, Gay, Bisexual, and Transgender (LGBT) Elders of Massachusetts: Focus on Home Care Study ($N = 76$)

Variable	%	Frequency
Sex/gender		
Female	90.8	69
Male	7.9	6
Transgender		
Male-to-female	0	0
Female-to-male	1.3	1
Race/ethnicity		
White/Caucasian	92.1	70
African American/Black	1.3	1
Asian/Asian American	2.6	2
Asian Pacific Islander	1.3	1
Cape Verdean	0	0
Haitian	0	0
Hispanic/Latino	0	0
Native American	1.3	1
Portuguese	0	0
Other	1.3	1
Sexual orientation		
Heterosexual	81.3	61
Gay/lesbian	13.3	10
Bisexual	5.3	4
Did not answer		1
Job classification		
Administrative support	0	0
Direct service	65	39
Manager/supervisor	35	21
Did not answer		16
Previous LGBT training		
Yes	38.7	29
No	61.3	46
Did not answer		1

White (70), two identified as Asian/Asian American, and one identified in each of the other categories of African American/Black, Pacific Islander, Native American, and other. Although age of the participant was not asked (an oversight in this research study), the majority of attendees were early to mid-career professionals with 39 working in direct service, 21 managers/supervisors, and 16 who did not answer. Most (46) had not previously received any training on LGBT awareness; 29 had attended a previous training on the topic. The providers identified primarily as heterosexual (61) with 14 identifying as LGBT, and one who did not answer.

Pretest and Posttest Comparison

Paired t tests were conducted to compare pre- and posttest scores on continuous measures. Results reported here are those with a significance level of $p < .001$ to control for Type I error (two-tailed); the complete list of comparisons appears in Table 2. Section A documented changes in provider attitudes by asking about participant feelings, including comfort in working with LGBT clients, disclosure issues, agency programs and same-sex spousal benefits. Of the 15 five-point questions asked, 10 showed statistically significant results using the more stringent alpha level. Results revealed a significant increase in awareness between pre- and posttest in knowledge about LGB resources, $t(76) = 7.854$, $p = .000$; transgender resources, $t(76) = 8.396$, $p = .000$; and policy disparities, $t(76) = 9.242$, $p = .000$. Participants' mean score between pre- and posttests also increased for the measures addressing whether "intake forms should include an opportunity to disclose sexual orientation and gender identity," $t(76) = 9.190$, $p = .000$; inquiring if "spousal benefits should be expanded for all," $t(76) = 5.232$, $p = .000$; knowing how to respond if an older adult came out as LGB, $t(76) = 4.312$, $p = .000$; and knowing how to respond if an older adult came out as transgender, $t(76) = 3.418$, $p = .000$. Finally, provider's mean score between pre- and posttests also increased when asked about their ability to help older adults who feel conflicted about being LGBT, $t(76) = 6.986$, $p = .000$; whether their agency should provide targeted services to LGBT older adults, $t(76) = 5.729$, $p = .000$; and if they (i.e., providers) felt that LGBT older adults face additional barriers to care compared to their heterosexual counterparts, $t(76) = 6.143$, $p = .000$.

Section C asked about what a participant "would" do in a specific situation to assess behavioral intentions. These responses may provide insight into whether an agency staff person was prepared to work effectively with LGBT clients and create an environment that was welcoming and safe. Only one of the four questions resulted in statistically significant differences. Provider's mean score between pre- and posttests increased with respect to challenging homophobic or transphobic remarks when heard, $t(76) = 3.559$ $p = .000$.

For pre- and posttest comparison of dichotomous questions, chi square analysis was used (see Table 3). Section B documented factual knowledge through seven true–false questions and one yes–no question. Of the eight questions, three resulted in significant differences in the pre- and posttest comparisons ($p < .001$). There was a significant improvement in factual knowledge level regarding homosexuality as a mental health diagnosis, $\chi^2 = 12.36$, $p = .000$; the Family and Medical Leave Act of 1993 (FMLA) policy on medical leave for same-sex couples, $\chi^2 = 24.68$, $p = .000$; and federal housing non-discrimination for sexual orientation, $\chi^2 = 42.39$, $p = .000$).

Supplemental Analyses

Supplemental analyses were conducted to test if the differences among the sexual orientation of the providers were significantly contributing to the results. Chi-square analyses were conducted to test for effects of sexual orientation. These analyses revealed that LGBT participants were significantly

TABLE 2 Pretest and Posttest Results of Study Participants in Lesbian, Gay, Bisexual, and Transgender (LGBT) Elders of Massachusetts: Focus on Home Care Study ($N = 76$).

Variable	Pretest		Posttest		
Survey Question	M	SD	M	SD	t
Section A					
Awareness of LGB resources	2.52	0.988	3.62	0.892	7.854***
Awareness of transgender resources	2.24	8.847	3.44	0.963	8.396***
Awareness of policy disparities	3.21	1.024	4.20	0.766	9.242***
Intake should include sexual orientation & gender identity disclosure	3.18	1.116	4.25	.0733	9.190***
Spousal benefits should be expanded for all	4.03	1.000	4.57	.0597	5.232***
I would know how to respond if an elder came out as LGB	3.65	0.878	4.08	.0731	4.312***
I would know how to respond if an elder came out as transgender	3.23	0.909	3.63	0.731	3.418***
I am comfortable in the home of an LGBT person	4.43	0.736	4.59	0.521	2.659**
I am comfortable providing services to an openly LGB elder	4.54	0.599	4.62	0.489	1.424
I am comfortable providing services to an openly transgender elder	4.18	0.795	4.13	0.640	−0.600
Each of us contributes to the homophobia in our society	3.67	0.949	3.84	0.901	1.889
I have the ability to help elders who feel conflicted about being LGBT	3.05	0.999	3.81	0.800	6.986***
My agency should provide services specially for LGBT elders	3.47	0.883	4.01	0.697	5.729***
I currently refer LGBT elders to appropriate support in the area	2.93	0.816	3.20	0.844	2.850**
LGBT elders face additional barriers to care than heterosexual peers	3.89	0.953	4.47	0.600	6.143***
Section B					
See Table 3					
Section C					
I think I can tell whether an elder is heterosexual or homosexual	2.57	0.774	2.67	0.741	1.409
I use inclusive words like partner and significant other	3.57	1.149	3.58	1.004	0.148
When I hear homophobic or transphobic jokes I challenge them	3.32	0.981	3.58	0.965	3.559***
I assume the elders I serve are heterosexual	2.97	1.09	3.00	1.139	0.241

**p < .01. ***p < .001 (two–tailed).

TABLE 3 Chi-Square Pretest and Posttest Analysis in Lesbian, Gay, Bisexual, and Transgender (LGBT) Elders of Massachusetts: Focus on Home Care Study ($N = 76$)

Section B: "True/Yes" Percentages	Pretest	Posttest	Chi-Square
LGBT elders do not have children	2.6	2.6	0
Life partners of LGBT persons are entitled to spousal social security	10.7	2.6	4.933*
LGBT elders have increased risk of untreated serious illness	65.8	92.1	4.381*
Homosexuality is a diagnosis of mental disorder in the *Diagnostic and Statistical Manual of Mental Disorders*	18.9	2.6	12.358***
Family and Medical Leave Act of 1993 requires unpaid leave to same-sex partner due to illness	40.8	6.6	24.676***
Federal housing mandate sexual orientation non-discrimination	74	13.2	42.393***
Same-sex partner pension and 401K are treated same as heterosexuals	8	0[1]	8**
I have objects in office that are welcoming environment for LGBT	28.4	33.8	0.469

*$p < .05$. **$p < .01$. ***$p < .001$ (two–tailed).

more likely than were the heterosexual respondents ($p < .05$) to agree with the following questions: "Intake forms should give the person the opportunity to disclose sexual orientation and gender identity," "I currently refer LGBT elders to appropriate support in my service area," "My agency should provide services specifically targeted to LGBT elders," "I know how to respond if an elder comes out as LGBT," "I am comfortable providing services to LGBT elders," "I am comfortable in the home of LGBT elders," and "I have the ability to help elders who feel conflicted about being LGBT." Analyses conducted excluding the LGBT participants, however, did not change the pattern of results already reported; that is, knowledge and attitudes increased significantly for both groups as a result of the intervention, notwithstanding higher values for the LGBT providers. As such, the simpler analyses are reported earlier.

An ANOVA was also conducted to test if there were differences between providers identifying as heterosexual and those identifying as LGBT in the pre- and posttest framework. On all comparisons, LGBT participants scored higher on both the pretest and the posttest compared to the heterosexual participants. The only interaction effects were noted on the questions addressing the awareness of LGB resources ($F = 4.963$, $p = .029$) and awareness of transgender resources ($F = 4.149$, $p = .046$) for which there were significant time by sexual orientation interactions. For these analyses, there was a greater increase in knowledge among the heterosexual identified participants. The fact that only two comparisons revealed significant interactions supports the previously mentioned findings of change over time

---

[1]Given the zero frequency in this cell, these computations must be treated with caution.

for providers, independent of sexual orientation. That is, the fact that there were LGBT providers as part of the sample did not drive the overall pattern of results; both groups increased in knowledge and attitudes as a consequence of this intervention.

DISCUSSION

This study was conducted to determine the impact and effectiveness of LGBT cultural competency training for mainstream elder service providers; the goal of this intervention was to improve provider awareness of the unique issues facing LGBT older adults and the professional capacity of agency personnel to serve their clients with dignity and respect. Analyses revealed statistically significant positive change in the knowledge, attitudes and behavioral intentions of the elder service providers who completed the LGBT aging training; LGBT cultural sensitivity trainings can effectuate positive change.

This study's findings indicated that an increased knowledge of public policies was particularly impactful in that all of the policy-related questions showed a statistically significant improvement suggesting that these trainings are effective in educating about current laws and disparities. For example, one item inquired if "The FMLA requires employers to grant unpaid leave of up to 12 weeks to an employee if their partner is ill, even if that employee's partner is of the same sex (true/false)"; at pretest, 59.2% answered correctly (i.e., noting that this statement was false), and at posttest that increased to 93.4% answering correctly. Many respondents' pretests overestimated LGBT inclusion in legal, financial, and health policies prior to the training and their posttest results reflected their increased knowledge of the lack of parity that exists in these areas. Many of these policies impact the services and benefits upon which clients might rely.

In addition to their improved familiarity with policy implications and disparities, participants also increased their awareness of resources for LGBT older adults and their families. Many of these participants function in roles that require them to provide information, referral, and resources to clients and their families. This training provided them with education and information that would increase their effectiveness in working with LGBT clients and was in keeping with other aspects of their continuing education and professional development.

Another facet of the training addressed participants' own attitudes toward LGBT issues in general and LGBT older adults in particular. Pretest results indicated that less than half of participants thought sexual orientation or gender identity should be included on initial intake forms. As previously discussed, the assumption by service providers that all older adults are heterosexual is widespread and results in minimizing the unique needs of LGBT older adults (AOA, 2010; Crisp, 2006; Turner et al., 2006). Although associated with risks and fears of discrimination (Johnson et al., 2005), disclosure of sexual orientation and gender identity by LGBT older adults is also credited with creating "more open and trusting relationships" with providers (IOM, 2011, p. 276; Orel, 2006). After the training, and with greater sensitivity of how important self-disclosure and visibility can be, participants who agreed/strongly agreed that the intake form should ask about sexual orientation and gender identity increased from 43.4% to 88.2%. If operationalized at the agency level, this change has the potential to lessen perceptions that providers are not sensitive to their needs (Butler, 2004; IOM, 2011). In addition, in Meyer's (2003) model, minority stress generates an internal anxiety that influences the decisions not to disclose; thus, if disclosure was alleviated at the onset, it may ease the resultant minority stress. The training also amplified respondents' understanding of how LGBT specific programming could be beneficial, as seen in an increase of support for LGBT programs.

Finally, the training highlighted participants' behavioral intentions and how they would expect to work with LGBT clients. Attendees reported increased confidence in their own abilities to challenge homophobic/transphobic remarks and to advocate for respectful environments. Given that Fairchild et al. (1996) found that half of nursing home direct-care staff made anti-gay comments and O'Hanlan et al. (1997) found the same among medical providers, a provider's ability to challenge such remarks could encourage culture change. They also reported increased comfort in their own ability to respond to clients who might come out to them about their sexual orientation. The distinction between participants' greater comfort in responding to sexual orientation versus gender identity is consistent with the broader culture's greater comfort level and exposure to more lesbian, gay, bisexual persons and less with transgender persons who remain invisible (Witten & Eyler, 2012). Of note, although not a significant finding, "I am comfortable providing services to an openly transgender elder" was the only question of the 32 in which providers showed a decrease in comfort level from the pretest to the posttest. One potential explanation may be that as providers learned more about the needs of transgender older adults, their confidence in their ability to meet those needs decreased.

Although a limitation of this study is the lack of demographic diversity among study participants, training attendees were both heterosexual and LGBT. Chi-square results showed that LGBT participants were significantly more likely to show high levels of comfort in working with LGBT elders; this would be expected as the LGBT community has a long history of caring for its own. A unique finding revealed in repeat measure analysis was that both heterosexual and LGBT participants showed increase posttest results in all questions. There was only one significant difference between the groups; a significant interaction between sexual orientation and awareness of LGBT resources showed a greater increase in knowledge among the heterosexual identified participants. This would be expected as the LGBT participants starting knowledge was much higher therefore there was less of a learning curve to attain.

Creating Change From Results

These survey results from four separate agencies indicate that mainstream elder service providers are receptive to improving their knowledge about LGBT older adults, expanding how they think about issues relating to LGBT older adults, and broadening how they intended to behave and interact with LGBT clients. The pre- and posttest data indicate that this one-time only training showed beneficial results regarding work with LGBT older adults. These positive results encouraged the expansion of these trainings to additional aging service agencies throughout the state network. Subsequent trainings at additional locations broadened the range of providers who could benefit from LGBT cultural competency training throughout the state of Massachusetts, thus increasing the inclusive services available to LGBT older adults statewide.

These pilot trainings were revised and incorporated into the LGBT Aging Project's LGBT Cultural Competency Training for Mainstream Elder Service Providers, known as The Open Door Task Force. Open Door's goal—to increase the professional capacity of mainstream elder service providers to serve LGBT clients—incorporated many of the elements of the pilot training. Open Door sought to increase knowledge of issues unique to LGBT older adults, improve participants' sensitivity toward such issues, and, generate action items that would create welcoming environments and programs for LGBT older adults and caregivers. The Open Door project expanded on the initial 1-day training session by adding a task force component; each organization convened an ad hoc work group that met with the trainer for a number of sessions over a period of months. These technical assistance sessions focused on how to institutionalize the organizations' commitment to creating a welcoming environment for LGBT older adults. This was achieved through the development of policies and procedures that are inclusive of LGBT clients, caregivers and staff; development of staff practice skills to implement LGBT inclusive policies; and communicating with community partners, along with current and potential clients, that the organization has a sustained commitment to the inclusion of LGBT clients, caregivers, and staff.

Landers, Mimiaga, and Krinsky (2010) conducted a qualitative study of Open Door in its earliest stages (2005–2007) and reported that participating agencies made policy changes, implemented staff training, and began developing programs and outreach to LGBT older adults and caregivers. Most respondents indicated that their organization's commitment to, and participation in, Open Door yielded increased recognition and normalization of LGBT issues in their agencies. In addition, Massachusetts's 2004 legalization of same-sex marriage, and subsequent legal appeals, brought LGBT issues to the general public's consciousness and the implications of marriage equality were considered in many arenas, including elder services. Some agencies incorporated Open Door's message of LGBT inclusion into their ongoing diversity efforts and others used it as a starting point for addressing inclusion of other less dominant populations they serve (Landers et al., 2010).

The paucity of available data showing the efficacy of LGBT aging awareness training programs has been a roadblock to funding for this type of education. This current study's pre- and posttest data has been used to effectively advocate to both funders and to elder service providers the positive impact of investing in such training. Nationwide data regarding the effectiveness and impact of LGBT cultural awareness training for mainstream elder services would be helpful to test the training among more diverse demographic participants of different urban and rural communities. Additional data is needed to support further expansion of such trainings throughout the elder care system and could support public and private funding to implement such trainings system wide.

Limitations

This study was limited by its quasi-experimental design, which included the absence of a control group. Given the disproportionate heterosexual orientation of the sample, the numbers were insufficient to make a fully adequate comparison between the heterosexual and the LGBT participants. The overall sample included both women and men; however, the numbers were insufficient to compare the genders on the dependent measures. Further limitations derive from the fact that participation was voluntary; therefore, it may indicate a greater interest or comfort level with the subject matter at baseline, thereby excluding the experiences of others with more profound opposition to the subject. Social desirability bias cannot be discounted from posttest results; however, the potential for this bias is reduced by the anonymity of the testing procedures and self-administered design. Notwithstanding these limitations and given how little research exists on this topic, this study serves as an important starting point and contribution to the dialogue.

Recommendations

LGBT cultural competency trainings for mainstream elder service providers have maintained their focus on three important areas: knowledge of unique factors for LGBT older adult, reflection on participants' attitudes about LGBT issues, and behavioral intentions in working with this population. The 1-day training sessions raised many important issues and potential action items for individuals and organizations to consider. The posttest data suggests the LGBT cultural competence training had a positive short-term impact on service providers; a follow-up evaluation to determine how well those changes were implemented without further reinforcement or encouragement is recommended. Reevaluating knowledge, attitudes, and behavioral intentions regarding work with LGBT clients at intervals of 3, 6, and 12 months, for example, might yield greater appreciation of the long term impact of the training.

Further evaluation is needed to revisit those agencies that participated in the early trainings (2003–2007) to assess long-term impact of these sessions. Topics for investigation include individual practice and organizational policies, how many LGBT older adults are served by these agencies, and any client impressions of change at the agency. Given the cultural changes that have occurred over the past decade (marriage equality in Massachusetts in 2004 and elsewhere in the country; state and federal policy recognition of LGBTs and their relationships) knowledge, attitudes and behavioral intention may have changed even more than initially reported.

In addition, an agency-level survey is recommended to appraise institutional change in culture as operationalized through policy and procedures. It is necessary to determine if the organization is committed to culture change and highlight any barriers that may inhibit such change. Organizations can create safe and welcoming environments for both staff and clients in various ways that include: revised nondiscrimination policies that provide inclusion of LGBT language, LGBT-specific programming, staff domestic partnership benefits, and FMLA protections for same-sex couples. Finally, changing attitudes may be an iterative process, therefore supplementary trainings may be recommended to elicit the sought after behavioral change.

The training showed particular strength in providing knowledge about existing resources and policies and that should continue to be a cornerstone of the training curriculum. Additional content related to transgender experiences may be helpful given this area showed a decreased comfort level. These data were limited demographically as participants were largely female, White, and heterosexual, so testing the curriculum with a more diversified participant base is recommended.

The Open Door Task Force, which was developed as a result of the pilot training programs described here, utilized the recommendation that culture change requires more than a single training session and, thus, incorporated ongoing consultation sessions over time to build each organization's sustainable commitment to LGBT inclusion. Landers et al. (2010) conducted their qualitative study when participating agencies were part way through the Open Door training. To evaluate the long term impact of participation in Open Door, those agencies should be revisited to assess their current policies, training, programs and commitment to LGBT inclusion as well as their ability to report how many LGBT clients and caregivers they have engaged with since participating in Open Door.

LGBT older adults, as is true of all older adults, deserve high quality, culturally competent aging and health related services. This study concludes that LGBT cultural sensitivity trainings for mainstream elder service providers can effectuate short term positive change in knowledge, attitudes, and behavior intentions. Further research is needed to evaluate the longer term impact of these efforts and implications for providers and the LGBT older adults and caregivers they serve.

FUNDING

The initial project for this study was funded by The Medical Foundation/ Farnsworth Trust.

REFERENCES

Administration on Aging. (2010). *LGBT elders technical assistance resources, 2010.* Washington, DC: Department of Health and Human Services. Retrieved from http://www.aoa.gov/AoARoot/Grants/Funding/docs/2010/-FINAL_LGBT_Elders_TA_Resource_Ctr.pdf

Bell, S. A., Bern-Klug, M., Kramer, K. W., & Saunders, J. B. (2010). Most nursing home social service directors lack training in working with lesbian, gay, and bisexual residents. *Social Work in Health Care, 49,* 814–831. doi:10.1080/00981389.2010.494561

Brotman, S., Cormier, R., & Ryan, B. (2001). The marginalization of gay and lesbian seniors in eldercare services. *Vital Aging, 7*(3), 2.

Butler, S. S. (2004). Gay, lesbian, bisexual, and transgender (GLBT) elders. *Journal of Human Behavior in the Social Environment, 9*(4), 25–44.

Cahill, S., & South, K. (2002). Policy issues affecting lesbian, gay, bisexual, and transgender people in retirement. *Generations, 26*(2), 49–54.

Clark, M. E., Landers, S., Linde, R., & Sperber, J. (2001). The GLBT health access project: A state-funded effort to improve access to care. *American Journal of Public Health, 91,* 895.

Connolly, L. (1996). Long-term care and hospice. *Journal of Gay & Lesbian Social Services, 5*(1), 77–92.

Crandall, S. J., George, G., Marion, G. S., & Davis, S. (2003). Applying theory to the design of cultural competency training for medical students: A case study. *Academic Medicine, 78,* 588.

Crisp, C. (2006). The Gay Affirmative Practice Scale (GAP): A new measure for assessing cultural competence with gay and lesbian clients. *Social Work, 51,* 115–126.

Crosson, J. C., Deng, W., Brazeau, C., Boyd, L., & Soto-Greene, M. (2004). Evaluating the effect of cultural competency training on medical student attitudes. *Family Medicine–Kansas City, 36,* 199–203.

Fairchild, S. K., Carrino, G. E., & Ramirez, M. (1996). Social workers' perceptions of staff attitudes toward resident sexuality in a random sample of New York state nursing homes. *Journal of Gerontological Social Work, 26*(1), 153–169.

Fredriksen-Goldsen, K., Kim, H., Emlet, C., Muraco, A., Erosheva, E., Hoy-Ellis, C., . . . Petry, H. (2011). *The aging and health report: disparities and resilience among lesbian, gay, bisexual and transgender older adults.* Seattle, WA: Institute for Multigenerational Health.

Grant, J. M., Koskovich, G., Frazer, M. S., & Bjerk, S. (2010). *Outing age 2010: Public policy issues affecting gay, lesbian, bisexual and transgender elders*. Washington, DC: National Gay and Lesbian Task Force.

Hinrichs, K. L. M., & Vacha-Haase, T. (2010). Staff perceptions of same-gender sexual contacts in long-term care facilities. *Journal of Homosexuality*, *57*(6), 776–789.

Institute of Medicine. (2011). *The health of lesbian, gay, bisexual, and transgender people: Building a foundation for better understanding*. Washington, DC: National Academies Press.

Johnson, M. J., Jackson, N. C., Arnette, J. K., & Koffman, S. D. (2005). Gay and lesbian perceptions of discrimination in retirement care facilities. *Journal of Homosexuality*, *49*(2), 83–102.

John Snow Inc. Research and Training Institute. (2003). *Lesbian, gay, bisexual and transgender elders of Massachusetts: Focus on home care*. Unpublished manuscript.

Landers, S., Mimiaga, M. J., & Krinsky, L. (2010). The open door project task force: A qualitative study on LGBT aging. *Journal of Gay & Lesbian Social Services*, *22*, 316–336.

Link, B. G., & Phelan, J. C. (2001). Conceptualizing stigma. *Annual Review of Sociology*, *27*, 363–385.

Mayer, K. H., Bradford, J. B., Makadon, H. J., Stall, R., Goldhammer, H., & Landers, S. (2008). Sexual and gender minority health: What we know and what needs to be done. *American Journal of Public Health*, *98*, 989.

MetLife Mature Market Institute. (2010). *Still out, still aging: The MetLife study of lesbian, gay, bisexual, and transgender baby boomers*. Westport, CT: Author.

Meyer, I. H. (2003). Prejudice, social stress, and mental health in lesbian, gay, and bisexual populations: Conceptual issues and research evidence. *Psychological Bulletin*, *129*, 674.

Morrow, D. (2001). Older gays and lesbians: Surviving a generation of hate and violence. *Journal of Gay & Lesbian Social Services*, *13*, 151–169.

National Senior Citizens Law Center. (2011). *LGBT older adults in long-term care facilities: Stories from the field*. Washington, DC: Author.

O'Hanlan, K. A., Cabaj, R. P., Schatz, B., Lock, J., & Nemrow, P. (1997). A review of the medical consequences of homophobia with suggestions for resolution. *Journal of the Gay and Lesbian Medical Association*, *1*(1), 25–39.

Orel, N. (2006). Community needs assessment: Documenting the need for affirmative services for LGB older adults. In D. Kimmel, T. Rose, & S. David (Eds.), *Lesbian, gay, bisexual, and transgender aging: Research and clinical perspectives* (pp. 227–246). New York, NY: Columbia University Press.

Shankle, M. D., Maxwell, C. A., Katzman, E. S., & Landers, S. (2003). An invisible population: Older lesbian, gay, bisexual, and transgender individuals. *Clinical Research and Regulatory Affairs*, *20*, 159–182.

Stein, G. L., Beckerman, N. L., & Sherman, P. A. (2010). Lesbian and gay elders and long-term care: Identifying the unique psychosocial perspectives and challenges. *Journal of Gerontological Social Work*, *53*, 421–435.

Turner, K. L., Wilson, W. L., & Shirah, M. K. (2006). Lesbian, gay, bisexual, and transgender cultural competency for public health practitioners. In M.D. Shankle (Ed.), *The handbook of lesbian, gay, bisexual, and transgender public health:*

A practitioner's guide to service (pp. 59–83). Binghamton, NY: Harrington Park Press.

Van Den Bergh, N., & Crisp, C. (2004). Defining culturally competent practice with sexual minorities: Implications for social work education and practice. *Journal of Social Work Education, 40*, 221–238.

Witten, T. M., & Eyler, A. E. (Eds.). (2012). *Gay, lesbian, bisexual and transgender aging: Challenges in research practice and policy.* Baltimore, MD: Johns Hopkins University Press.

Index

Page numbers in bold refer to figures or tables